T0226954

Screening and Prevention in Geriatric Medicine

Editors

DANELLE CAYEA
SAMUEL C. DURSO

CLINICS IN GERIATRIC MEDICINE

www.geriatric.theclinics.com

February 2018 • Volume 34 • Number 1

ELSEVIER

1600 John F. Kennedy Boulevard • Suite 1800 • Philadelphia, Pennsylvania, 19103-2899

http://www.theclinics.com

CLINICS IN GERIATRIC MEDICINE Volume 34, Number 1
February 2018 ISSN 0749–0690, ISBN-13: 978-0-323-56980-4

Editor: Jessica McCool
Developmental Editor: Laura Fisher

Clinics in Geriatric Medicine (ISSN 0749-0690) is published quarterly by Elsevier Inc., 360 Park Avenue South, New York, NY 10010-1710. Months of issue are February, May, August, and November. Business and Editorial Offices: 1600 John F. Kennedy Blvd., Suite 1800, Philadelphia, PA 191023-2899. Periodicals postage paid at New York, NY, and additional mailing offices. Subscription prices are $278.00 per year (US individuals), $602.00 per year (US institutions), $100.00 per year (US student/resident), $320.00 per year (Canadian individuals), $763.00 per year (Canadian institutions), $195.00 per year (Canadian student/resident), $402.00 per year (international individuals), $763.00 per year (international institutions), and $195.00 per year (international student/resident). Foreign air speed delivery is included in all *Clinics* subscription prices. All prices are subject to change without notice. POSTMASTER: Send address changes to *Clinics in Geriatric Medicine,* Elsevier Health Sciences Division, Subscription Customer Service, 3251 Riverport Lane, Maryland Heights, MO 63043. **Telephone: 1-800-654-2452 (U.S. and Canada); 314-447-8871 (outside U.S. and Canada). Fax: 314-447-8029. E-mail:** journalscustomerservice-usa@elsevier. com **(for print support) or** journalsonlinesupport-usa@elsevier.com **(for online support).**

Reprints. For copies of 100 or more, of articles in this publication, please contact the Commercial Reprints Department, Elsevier Inc., 360 Park Avenue South, New York, New York 10010-1710. Tel.: 212-633-3874; Fax: 212-633-3820, E-mail: reprints@elsevier.com.

Clinics in Geriatric Medicine is covered in *MEDLINE/PubMed (Index Medicus), EMBASE/Excerpta Medica, Current Contents/Clinical Medicine (CC/CM),* and the *Cumulative Index to Nursing & Allied Health Literature.*

Contributors

EDITORS

DANELLE CAYEA, MD, MS
Associate Professor of Medicine, Director, Daniel and Jeanette Hendin Schapiro Geriatric Medical Education Center, Division of Geriatric Medicine and Gerontology, The Johns Hopkins University School of Medicine, Baltimore, Maryland

SAMUEL C. DURSO, MD, MBA
Mason F. Lord Professor of Medicine, Division of Geriatric Medicine and Gerontology, The Johns Hopkins University School of Medicine, Baltimore, Maryland

AUTHORS

MEGAN BURKE, MD
Postdoctoral Fellow, Geriatric Medicine and Gerontology, The Johns Hopkins University School of Medicine, Johns Hopkins Bayview Medical Center, Baltimore, Maryland

BRIAN BUTA, MHS
Claude D. Pepper Older Americans Independence Center, Johns Hopkins University, Division of Geriatric Medicine and Gerontology, Center on Aging and Health, The Johns Hopkins University School of Medicine, Baltimore, Maryland

MIRNOVA E. CEÏDE, MD
Assistant Professor, Divisions of Geriatric Psychiatry and Geriatric Medicine, Departments of Psychiatry and Behavioral Science and Internal Medicine, Montefiore Medical Center, Albert Einstein College of Medicine, Bronx, New York

JESSICA L. COLBURN, MD
Assistant Professor of Medicine, Divisions of Geriatric Medicine and Gerontology and General Internal Medicine, The Johns Hopkins University School of Medicine, Baltimore, Maryland

SHELLY L. GRAY, PharmD, MS
Professor, Department of Pharmacy, University of Washington, School of Pharmacy, Seattle, Washington

BENJAMIN H. HAN, MD, MPH
Assistant Professor, Division of Geriatric Medicine and Palliative Care, Department of Medicine, NYU School of Medicine, New York, New York

RUSSELL P. HARRIS, MD, MPH
Emeritus Professor of Medicine, Division of General Medicine and Clinical Epidemiology, Sheps Center for Health Services Research, The University of North Carolina at Chapel Hill, Chapel Hill, North Carolina

MITCHELL T. HEFLIN, MD, MHS
Associate Professor of Medicine, Division of Geriatrics, Duke University School of Medicine, Durham, North Carolina

HOLLY M. HOLMES, MD, MS
Associate Professor and Division Director, Division of Geriatric and Palliative Medicine, The University of Texas Health Science Center at Houston, McGovern Medical School, Houston, Texas

GARY J. KENNEDY, MD
Vice Chair for Education, Professor, and Director, Division of Geriatric Psychiatry, Department of Psychiatry and Behavioral Science, Montefiore Medical Center, Albert Einstein College of Medicine, Bronx, New York

KIMBERLEY T. LEE, MD
Clinical Fellow, Division of Oncology, Department of Medicine, The Johns Hopkins University School of Medicine, Baltimore, Maryland

ZACHARY A. MARCUM, PharmD, PhD
Assistant Professor, Department of Pharmacy, University of Washington, School of Pharmacy, Seattle, Washington

JULIANNA G. MARWELL, MD
Assistant Professor, Department of Medicine, The Medical University of South Carolina, Charleston, South Carolina

SHELLEY R. McDONALD, DO, PhD
Assistant Professor of Medicine, Division of Geriatrics, Duke University School of Medicine, Durham, North Carolina

ALISON A. MOORE, MD, MPH
Professor of Medicine, Chief of Geriatric Medicine, UC San Diego School of Medicine, La Jolla, California

JORGE CAMILO MORA, MD, MPH
Director of Geriatric Medicine, Leader of the Professional Development Curricular Strand, Director of Clinical Nutrition, FIU Herbert Wertheim College of Medicine, Miami, Florida

EMILY MORGAN, MD
Assistant Professor of Medicine, Division of Internal Medicine and Geriatrics, Oregon Health and Science University, Portland, Oregon

STEPHANIE NOTHELLE, MD
Postdoctoral Fellow, Divisions of Geriatric Medicine and Gerontology and General Internal Medicine, The Johns Hopkins University School of Medicine, Baltimore, Maryland

ARIELA R. ORKABY, MD, MPH
Geriatrician, Preventive Cardiology, Geriatric Research, Education, and Clinical Center (GRECC), VA Boston Healthcare System, Instructor, Medicine, Associate Epidemiologist, Division of Aging, Brigham and Women's Hospital, Harvard Medical School, Boston, Massachusetts

MICHAEL W. RICH, MD, FACC, AGSF
Professor of Medicine, Washington University School of Medicine in St. Louis, St Louis, Missouri

THERESA ROWE, DO, MS
Assistant Professor, General Internal Medicine and Geriatrics, Northwestern University Feinberg School of Medicine, Chicago, Illinois

NANCY L. SCHOENBORN, MD
Assistant Professor, Division of Geriatric Medicine and Gerontology, Department of Medicine, The Johns Hopkins University School of Medicine, Baltimore, Maryland

AMIT A. SHAH, MD
Department of Internal Medicine, Mayo Clinic, Scottsdale, Arizona

ERIN M. SMITH, MD
Department of Internal Medicine, Mayo Clinic, Scottsdale, Arizona

WILLY M. VALENCIA, MD
Voluntary Assistant Professor, Department of Public Health Sciences, ABIM Internal Medicine, Geriatric Medicine, Endocrinology, Diabetes & Metabolism Full-time Physician Scientist, Miami VA Healthcare System, Geriatrics Research, Education & Clinical Center (GRECC), University of Miami Miller School of Medicine, Miami, Florida

JEREMY WALSTON, MD
Claude D. Pepper Older Americans Independence Center, Johns Hopkins University, Division of Geriatric Medicine and Gerontology, Center on Aging and Health, The Johns Hopkins University School of Medicine, Baltimore, Maryland

QIAN-LI XUE, PhD
Claude D. Pepper Older Americans Independence Center, Johns Hopkins University, Division of Geriatric Medicine and Gerontology, Center on Aging and Health, The Johns Hopkins University School of Medicine, Baltimore, Maryland

ANDREW R. ZULLO, PharmD, PhD
Assistant Professor, Department of Health Services, Policy, and Practice, The School of Public Health at Brown University, Providence, Rhode Island

Contents

overwhelming, but starting with a focused approach and leveraging a team-based strategy can help practicing clinicians gain initial momentum. Future research is needed to strengthen the evidence base for medication use in older adults and to elucidate effective and scalable interventions to improve medication safety.

The geriatric syndromes of falls, incontinence, and osteoporosis are concerns in older adults because of their potential impact on quality of life. Asking about history of falls or a fear of falling should prompt a multifactorial assessment of fall risk and targeted interventions to reduce falls. Urinary and fecal incontinence should be screened because they are common conditions that are underreported because of embarrassment and general perception that incontinence is a normal part of aging. Women older than 65 years, men older than 70 years, and younger patients with high-risk characteristics should be screened with bone mineral density testing with dual-energy x-ray absorptiometry.

Avoidable disability associated with depression, anxiety, and impaired cognition among older adults is pervasive. Incentives for detection of mental disorders in late life include increased reimbursement, reduced cost, and less burden for patients and families. However, screening not aligned with diagnosis, intervention, and outcome assessment has questionable utility. The link between screening, treatment, and outcomes is well established for depression, less so for anxiety and impaired cognition. This article details the use of common instruments to screen and assess depression, anxiety, and cognitive impairment.

Evidence for preventive screening and therapeutic intervention for primary prevention of cardiovascular disease is limited for older adults. This article reviews screening and prevention strategies, including lifestyle, modifiable risk factors, and medications, that may be considered in older adults, with a focus on those 75 years or older, accounting for age, frailty and functional status, medical conditions, and life expectancy.

Older adults undergoing elective surgical procedures suffer higher rates of morbidity and mortality than younger patients. A geriatric-focused preoperative evaluation can identify risk factors for complications and opportunities for health optimization and care coordination. Key components of a geriatric preoperative evaluation include (1) assessments of function, mobility, cognition, and mental health; (2) reviews of medical conditions and medications; and (3) discussion of risks, preferences, and goals of care. A geriatric-focused, team-based approach can improve surgical outcomes and patient experience.

Emily Morgan

Clinical assessment of fitness to drive can be a challenging part of primary care of older adults. There are no guidelines on screening for driver safety, so it falls to provider judgment on when to assess older drivers. This article offers recommendations on when to assess for driver safety based on red flag conditions, medications, acute events, and patient or family concerns. It reviews how to assess for visual, cognitive, and neuromuscular impairments and what to do as next steps for at-risk drivers once they are identified. Laws regarding driver reporting are also reviewed.

Benjamin H. Han and Alison A. Moore

The number of older adults who engage in unhealthy substance use is expected to increase substantially to levels never seen before. Older adults, owing to physiologic changes in aging, are at high risk for the adverse effects of alcohol and illegal drug use. Screening and prevention can help older patients to be better informed of the risks of substance use and reduce high-risk behaviors and its potential negative outcomes. The authors review the prevalence and trends of substance use and the potential impact on health outcomes and discuss an approach to screening and prevention for older adults.

Megan Burke and Theresa Rowe

Vaccines are important for preventing infections in adults 65 years or older. Older adults are at increased risk for complications from vaccine-preventable illnesses because of age-associated changes in immune function and chronic medical comorbidities. Vaccination rates for older adults remain low despite widely accepted practice guidelines. Recommended vaccinations for older adults include (1) influenza; (2) pneumococcal; (3) herpes zoster; (4) tetanus, diphtheria, pertussis; and (5) hepatitis B. Cost influences vaccination rates in older adults.

Jorge Camilo Mora and Willy M. Valencia

Regular exercise is essential for healthy aging and offers many health benefits, including reduced risk of all-cause mortality, chronic disease, and premature death. Because physical inactivity is prevalent, greater focus is needed on integrating exercise into care plans and counseling and developing partnerships that support exercise opportunities. Older adults should be as physically active as their abilities and conditions allow. For substantial health benefits, older adults need to do aerobic, muscle-strengthening, and stretching exercises weekly and balance activities as needed. Appropriate planning must take account of factors such as prescribed medications, nutrition, injuries, hip and knee arthroplasties, and chronic conditions.

CLINICS IN GERIATRIC MEDICINE

ISSUE OF RELATED INTEREST

Medical Clinics, July 2017 (Vol. 101, No. 4)
Disease Prevention
Michael P. Pignone and Kirsten Bibbins-Domingo, *Editors*
http://www.medical.theclinics.com

THE CLINICS ARE AVAILABLE ONLINE!
Access your subscription at:
www.theclinics.com

CLINICS IN GERIATRIC MEDICINE

Preface

Screening and Prevention in the Modern Era

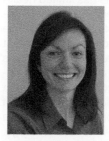 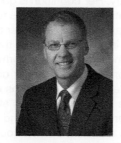

Danelle Cayea, MD, MS   Samuel C. Durso, MD, MBA
Editors

Prevention and early detection of treatable medical conditions is an appealing concept. Preventive health care encompasses primary prevention of illness (eg, immunization against infectious disease or adoption of a healthy lifestyle), secondary prevention that involves early detection of latent disease (eg, colon and breast cancer screening), or tertiary prevention that aims to limit disability or improve function for an individual with an existing condition (eg, exercise rehabilitation in chronic lung disease). Positioned at the interface between public health and individual medical care, preventive health care is implemented at the population level as well as at the individual level in the health care setting. The focus of these articles is care of the individual geriatric patient.

As with so much of geriatric medical care, the promise of prevention and screening is complicated. For example, the evidence base supporting most commonly accepted recommendations for primary and secondary preventive health care rarely includes adults over the age of 75 or those with multiple chronic illnesses or frailty. Preventive health care in the busy practice setting is challenging as it frequently competes for time needed to manage acute and chronic conditions. Furthermore, implementation requires a nuanced approach that considers the individual's health and function, life expectancy, and goals of care (eg, symptom management, preservation of function, or maximum longevity), while judging benefit and harm that is frequently not quantifiable. All of this must be communicated in a way that is considerate of health literacy and beliefs, sensory limitations, and cognitive function and may involve caregivers.

Disclosure: Dr D. Cayea is supported by the Daniel and Jeanette Hendin Schapiro Geriatric Medical Education Center.

Clin Geriatr Med 34 (2018) xiii–xvii
https://doi.org/10.1016/j.cger.2017.09.007
0749-0690/18/© 2017 Published by Elsevier Inc.

For example, consider a 75-year-old woman with intermittently symptomatic chronic obstructive lung disease, hypertension, and osteoporosis. She lives with her husband, who has early Alzheimer dementia. Although her mood is fine, she sometimes feels overwhelmed by his dependency on her. She is functionally independent within the home, but requires assistance with transportation. She and her husband experience moderate financial stress, but they do own a computer. An initial 1-hour physician office visit finds that her blood pressure is higher than recommended, and she has hearing loss and gait instability. Her cognition is good. She has limited health literacy, specifically relating to preventive health care. She received a 23-valent pneumococcal vaccine more than a decade ago, but no longer accepts influenza vaccine since she developed a respiratory infection following the injection. She has not received other recommended vaccines. She had a normal mammogram 2 years ago, but has never been screened for colon cancer. Her diet is relatively high in sodium, low in calcium and fiber. There are literally dozens of recommendations that could be characterized as preventive health care. She is at risk for complications of hypertension, respiratory infection, and injurious falls and osteoporotic fractures in addition to many more vulnerabilities and conditions associated with advanced age. Where does one start to counsel her?

Ideally, her physician will want to appreciate her intermediate and long-term goals of care. She will need to assess her willingness and capacity for change. The physician will also need to have a sense of the value of various interventions in order to prioritize and advise the patient. The patient will need enough knowledge to make informed choices and adhere to care plans, as well as necessary financial resources. Both the patient and the physician need information and payment systems to support their prevention efforts. Preventive health care in the 21st century offers some solutions to these issues, but also presents some challenges and leaves questions unanswered.

Commonly, older patients visit their physicians to discuss chronic conditions. Primary care doctors need to look for opportunities to implement preventive health care and educate patients in the midst of managing chronic conditions, which can be difficult. The Patient Protection and Affordable Care Act requires private insurance companies to cover recommended preventive services without patient cost-sharing. This led to the creation of the Annual Wellness Visit (AWV) benefit for Medicare recipients in 2011.[1] If our patient is able to return for a separate AWV, her physician could spend dedicated time discussing some of her unique preventive health care concerns, without placing financial burden on her or the physician. Depending on her preferences, this may afford her physician the time to discuss immunizations, individualized cancer screening, and fall risk. Thus far, the AWV has significantly increased rates of preventive services visits (1.4% to 27.5%) among Medicare fee-for-service beneficiaries, primarily among younger older adults with fewer chronic health conditions, but is still underutilized overall.[1,2] The AWV has modestly increased rates of some preventive care services (mammography, advance directive discussion, abdominal aortic aneurysm screening), but has been less effective in increasing rates of other services (depression screening, bone densitometry, colorectal cancer screening).[1,3,4]

While the AWV has increased rates of preventive services uptake, it is less well known whether the benefits outweigh the risks of the services used by individual patients. Predicting the relative value of a test or treatment for an individual requires combining knowledge of the patient's health status, estimated prognosis, potential benefits and harms of specific tests or treatments, and the patient's values and preferences. Our patient may prioritize interventions that maintain her functional independence and provide short- to medium-term benefit. The US Preventive Services Task Force recommends a framework for individualizing cancer screening for older adults.[5]

Understanding patients' preferences and goals is an essential element of having these discussions. Incorporating prognosis information in conversations with patients can be difficult for both the patient and the physician. Busy clinicians may be aided in these discussions by combining tools to measure prognosis with clinical judgment and decision aids to help patients understand these complex decisions.[6] Decision aids have been shown to increase patients' knowledge and reduce decisional conflict. There are a growing number of aids available to guide screening decisions for older adults.[7,8]

The explosion of technology and patients' ability to access it offers opportunities for increasing patients' health literacy and health management. As part of the AWV, the physician may ask the patient to read information to aid decision-making online. A wealth of health information is available on the Internet. When directed to high-quality sites, patients may use this information to better guide discussion with their physicians, decision making, and management of health.

Even when older adults have Internet access, accessing online health information is often challenging. These systems may not yet be optimized for use by all older adults, many of whom have lower numeracy and Internet experience, and current rates of adoption are low among older adults.[9] Older adults have difficulty completing simple and complex simulated tasks in a simulated online patient electronic health record (EHR) portal, with only 11.8% of all participants completing all of the simple tasks correctly.[10] There are numerous mobile health-related applications ("apps") available. To ensure successful use by older adults, apps must have design and functionality that adapt to sensory impairment, restricted range of finger motion from arthritis, and lower health literacy and possible cognitive impairment, among other considerations.[11] Even if our patient was not able to successfully navigate online health information, technology can help provide printed material to the patient. Some EHRs have options to include patient education in the after-visit summary. The National Institute on Aging has a library of high-quality fact sheets for patients, including several about caregiving, which may be helpful for our patient.[12]

During a follow-up visit, our patient's physician may be prompted by the EHR to complete several health maintenance activities. Health information technology and widespread implementation of the EHR provides opportunities and challenges in the practices of screening and disease prevention. Collation of data into one platform, computerized reminders and decision support tools, and integration with immunization information systems (IIS) make tracking of screening and immunizations much easier than before. All 50 states now have IIS in place, which allows for comprehensive immunization histories, regardless of provider, across time. Stage 3 of Meaningful Use for EHRs includes use of IIS clinical decision support for immunizations' functionality.[13] Computerized reminders moderately increase physicians' preventive care compliance (average difference 13%) and may be most effective for smoking cessation (average difference 23%) and cardiovascular screening (average difference 20%).[14] Ideally, our patient's record would only contain prompts for health maintenance activities that are likely to benefit her and consistent with her goals. The functionality of clinical decision support tools and EHR data analysis is expanding and improving. Frailty risk scores can be calculated for hospitalized patients using EHR clinical data, and future decision support tools may automate screening for frailty using EHR data.[15] Approximately 40% of the Assessing Care for Vulnerable Elders clinical rules can be automatically assessed using EHR data.[16]

However, older adults with multiple chronic conditions require individualized decisions about many screening tests, and algorithmic decision support tools in their current form may not be useful for those patients. A recent expert panel issued a consensus statement on measures of high-quality care for people with multiple chronic conditions, some of which are focused on appropriate use of screening and prevention, and noted that measurement would require adaptation of EHR technology.[17]

Continued improvements in disease and disability prevention will require coordinated efforts to increase patient engagement and community-clinic integration to increase access and delivery of services. The Centers for Disease Control and Prevention have laid a framework to accomplish this.[18] This issue of *Clinics in Geriatric Medicine* will cover many of the clinical, public health, and individual factors that lead to improved and appropriate delivery of preventive health care.

Danelle Cayea, MD, MS
Johns Hopkins University School of Medicine
Division of Geriatric Medicine and Gerontology
5500 Eastern Avenue
Mason F. Lord Building
Center Tower, Suite 2200, Room 208
Baltimore, MD 21224, USA

Samuel C. Durso, MD, MBA
Johns Hopkins University School of Medicine
Division of Geriatric Medicine and Gerontology
5200 Eastern Avenue
Mason F. Lord Building
Center Tower, Floor 3, DOM Suite, Room 317
Baltimore, MD 21224, USA

E-mail addresses:
dcayea1@jhmi.edu (D. Cayea)
sdurso@jhmi.edu (S.C. Durso)

REFERENCES

1. Chung S, Lesser LI, Lauderdale DS, et al. Medicare annual preventive care visits: use increased among fee-for-service patients, but many do not participate. Health Aff 2015;34:111–20.

2. Hu J, Jensen G, Nerenz D, et al. Medicare's annual wellness visit in a large health care organization: who is using it? Ann Intern Med 2015;163:567–8.

3. Cooper GS, Kou TD, Schluchter MD, et al. Changes in receipt of cancer screening in Medicare beneficiaries following the Affordable Care Act. J Natl Cancer Inst 2016;108(5):djv374.

4. Pfoh E, Mojtabai R, Bailey J, et al. Impact of Medicare annual wellness visits on uptake of depression screening. Psychiatr Serv 2015;66:1207–12.

5. Eckstrom E, Feeny DH, Walter LC, et al. Individualizing cancer screening in older adults: a narrative review and framework for future research. J Gen Intern Med 2013;28:292–8.

6. Lee S, Smith A, Widera E, et al. ePrognosis: estimating prognosis for elders. San Francisco (CA): University of California San Francisco; 2012. Available at: http://www.eprognosis.org. Accessed May 13, 2017.

7. Stacey D, Légaré F, Col NF, et al. Decision aids for people facing health treatment or screening decisions. Cochrane Database Syst Rev 2014;(1):CD001431.

8. Schonberg MA, Hamel MB, Davis RB, et al. Development and evaluation of a decision aid on mammography screening for women 75 years and older. JAMA Intern Med 2014;174:417–24.
9. Wildenbos GA, Peute L, Jaspers M. Facilitators and barriers of electronic health record patient portal adoption by older adults: a literature study. Stud Health Technol Inform 2017;235:308–12.
10. Taha J, Sharit J, Czaja SJ. The impact of numeracy ability and technology skills on older adults' performance of health management tasks using a patient portal. J Appl Gerontol 2014;33:416–36.
11. Wildenbos GA, Peute LW, Jaspers MW. A framework for evaluating mHealth tools for older patients on usability. Stud Health Technol Inform 2015;210:783–7.
12. National Institute of Aging. A-Z Health Topics Index. Available at: https://www.nia.nih.gov/health. Accessed June 12, 2017.
13. Centers for Disease Control and Prevention. Immunization Information Systems (IIS). 2014. Available at: http://www.cdc.gov.ezp.welch.jhmi.edu/vaccines/programs/iis/index.html. Accessed May 7, 2017.
14. Dexheimer JW, Talbot TR, Sanders DL, et al. Prompting clinicians about preventive care measures: a systematic review of randomized controlled trials. J Am Med Inform Assoc 2008;15:311–20.
15. Lekan DA, Wallace DC, McCoy TP, et al. Frailty assessment in hospitalized older adults using the electronic health record. Biol Res Nurs 2016;19:213–28.
16. Opondo D, Visscher S, Eslami S, et al. Feasibility of automatic evaluation of clinical rules in general practice. Int J Med Inform 2017;100:90–4.
17. Bayliss E, McQuillan DB, Ellis JL, et al. Using electronic health record data to measure care quality for individuals with multiple chronic medical conditions. J Am Geriatr Soc 2016;64:1839–44.
18. Krist A, Shenson D, Woolf S, et al. A framework for integration of community and clinical care to improve the delivery of clinical preventive services among older adults. A report prepared for the National Association of Chronic Disease Directors and the Michigan Public Health Institute, with funding provided by the Healthy Aging Program, Division of Population Health, Centers for Disease Control and Prevention July 2012. Available at: https://www.cdc.gov/aging/pdf/cps-integration-framework.pdf. Accessed June 12, 2017.

The Medicare Annual Wellness Visit

Jessica L. Colburn, MD[a],*, Stephanie Nothelle, MD[b]

KEYWORDS

- Medicare • Aged • Aged 80 and over • Geriatric assessment • Primary health care
- Preventive health services • Workflow

KEY POINTS

- The Medicare Annual Wellness Visit is an annual preventive health benefit covered by Medicare.
- The Annual Wellness Visit is an opportunity for physicians and teams to review geriatric syndromes and discuss goals with older adults.
- Physicians should consider preventive health recommendations in the context of a patient's goals of care and overall prognosis.
- Physicians and team members, including nurses and pharmacists, have several options for incorporating the Annual Wellness Visit into a busy clinic workflow.

INTRODUCTION

The Medicare Annual Wellness Visit (AWV) was created as part of the Patient Protection and Affordable Care Act in 2011 to expand coverage of preventive health care services to older adults. All Medicare beneficiaries who have been enrolled in Medicare Part B for 12 months are eligible for the AWV. Eligible beneficiaries can receive an initial AWV followed by a subsequent AWV every 12 months.

During the AWV, a clinician can step back from the visit-to-visit care and focus on the overall care plan, including preventive health, disease screening, and coordination of care. The patient completes a health risk assessment and receives a personalized prevention plan and appropriate referrals based on identified needs. This visit has the

Conflicts of Interest: None. No financial disclosures to report.
Funding Sources: Dr J.L. Colburn and S. Nothelle are supported by the Geriatrics Workforce Enhancement Program (U1QHP28710-02-00), provided by the Health Services Research Administration.
[a] Division of Geriatric Medicine and Gerontology, Johns Hopkins University School of Medicine, 5200 Eastern Avenue, Suite 2200, Baltimore, MD 21224, USA; [b] Division of Geriatric Medicine and Gerontology, Johns Hopkins University School of Medicine, 5200 Eastern Avenue, 7th Floor, Baltimore, MD 21224, USA
* Corresponding author.
E-mail address: jcolbur1@jhmi.edu

https://doi.org/10.1016/j.cger.2017.09.001
0749-0690/18/© 2017 Elsevier Inc. All rights reserved.
geriatric.theclinics.com

potential to be a geriatric assessment tool, given that many of the required components pertain to geriatric syndromes such as assessment of cognitive and functional status, screening for depression, and fall risk assessment. This screening provides an opportunity to assess whether the patient's care is matched to his/her goals, prognosis, and values.

The AWV is a co-pay–free visit for patients and is reimbursed at a higher rate than a typical office visit. Despite the potential incentives, it has not been widely adopted by primary care practices. Only 15% of eligible patients received the AWV in 2014, a rate that varied from 3% to 30% depending on the region of practice. Despite these low overall rates, close to half (40%) of primary care clinicians completed an AWV in 2014.[1]

ELEMENTS OF THE ANNUAL WELLNESS VISIT

The Center for Medicare and Medicaid Services (CMS) has specific requirements for elements that need to be included in the AWV.[2] The initial AWV and the subsequent AWV have different requirements, although practices may choose to approach the visit similarly in evaluation and workflow. **Table 1** lists the requirements for the initial and subsequent AWV. Additional information is available on www.cms.gov.

Table 1
Requirements of the initial and subsequent annual wellness visit

Required Elements	Initial AWV	Subsequent AWV
Health risk assessment (HRA)	X	X
Establish past medical & surgical history, family history, allergies	X	X
List of current providers and suppliers	X	X
List of current medications, including supplements	X	X
Patient assessment: height, weight, body mass index, blood pressure, other measurements as deemed appropriate (does not include a physical examination)	X	X
Screening for cognitive impairment	X	X
Screening for depression and risk factors for depression	X	
Screening for functional ability and safety, including hearing impairment, ability to perform ADLs, fall risk, home safety	X	
Provide the patient with a written screening schedule for appropriate preventive health services	X	Update of written screening schedule
Provide the patient with a list of risk factors and conditions for which interventions are recommended or underway	X	X
Provide the patient with personalized health advice for health education or lifestyle interventions (may include community resources)	X	X

Data from Centers for Medicare and Medicaid Services. The ABCs of the Annual Wellness Visit (AWV). https://www.cms.gov/Outreach-and-Education/Medicare-Learning-Network-MLN/MLNProducts/downloads/AWV_chart_ICN905706.pdf. Accessed June 12, 2017.

The Health Risk Assessment (HRA) is a required component of the AWV that provides an initial screening for a variety of geriatric syndromes and risk factors.[3] The HRA can be completed before the visit through the online patient portal of the electronic medical record or a paper form can be mailed to the patient. Alternatively, some practices choose to have the patient fill out the HRA form in the waiting room or have a medical assistant or the provider ask the questions directly during the visit. There are sample forms published online by various health systems, or some health systems choose to create their own HRA form, which can be incorporated into the electronic medical record. **Table 2** lists required components in the HRA form.

GERIATRIC ASSESSMENT IN THE ANNUAL WELLNESS VISIT

The HRA includes several questions about geriatric syndromes, which serve as basic screening tools. If the answer to any of the questions indicates an issue, such as falls or trouble with memory, the physician and clinic staff may elect to do additional testing and evaluation at the same visit (billed with a -25 modifier as a problem-based visit) or may schedule the patient to return for a follow-up visit.

Cognitive Screening

There is evidence that dementia is underdiagnosed in primary care, and that as many as 81% of patients who meet criteria for dementia have not received a formal diagnosis.[4] Identification of patients with cognitive impairment and dementia may help to connect patients and caregivers with education about the progression of dementia, community resources and support, and opportunities for advance care planning.

Cognitive screening is a required element of both the initial and the subsequent AWV. CMS does not require or recommend a specific screening tool or approach to screening. The Alzheimer's Association convened a workgroup to develop a recommended algorithm for primary care physicians to use for cognitive screening during the AWV.[5] The expert workgroup recommends beginning with HRA review, which should include specific questioning about confusion or memory loss in the past 12 months as well as assistance with activities of daily living (ADLs) or instrumental activities of daily living (IADLs). If the patient answers "yes" for memory loss, confusion, or need for assistance with ADLs or IADLs, the next step is to proceed with a brief structured assessment such as the Mini-Cog, General Practitioner Assessment of

Table 2 Health risk assessment requirements	
Category	**Specific Elements to be Included**
Demographic data	Age, gender, race, ethnicity
Self-assessment	Health status, frailty, physical functioning
Psychosocial risks	Depression, stress, anger, loneliness/social isolation, pain, fatigue
Behavioral risks	Smoking, physical activity, nutrition/oral health, alcohol use, sexual health, seat belt use, home safety
ADLs	Dressing, feeding, toileting, grooming, bathing, ambulation
IADLs	Shopping, food preparation, telephone, housekeeping, laundry, transportation, medications, finances

Data from Centers for Medicare and Medicaid Services. Frequently asked questions from the March 28, 2012 Medicare Preventive Services National Provider Call: the initial preventive physical exam and the Annual Wellness Visit. Available at: https://www.cms.gov/Outreach-and-Education/Outreach/NPC/Downloads/IPPE-AWV-FAQs.pdf. Accessed June 12, 2017.

Cognition, or Memory Impairment Screen,[6] and if positive, to proceed to a full dementia evaluation. If the patient and informant do not report any concerns about memory or functional impairment, then additional testing can be deferred, and it is recommended that the physician follow-up with screening at the subsequent AWV.

Dementia is a clinical diagnosis based on defined criteria and can be diagnosed in primary care by internists and family practitioners. The Diagnostic and Statistical Manual of Mental Disorders, Fifth Edition defines major neurocognitive disorder (previously called dementia) as:

- Evidence of significant cognitive decline from a previous level of performance in one or more cognitive domains: learning and memory, language, executive function, complex attention, perceptual-motor, or social cognition;
- Interference of cognitive deficits with independence in everyday activities (at a minimum, interference with complex IADL, such as paying bills or managing medications);
- Cognitive deficits that do not occur exclusively due to delirium; and cognitive deficits that are not explained by another mental disorder such as major depressive disorder or schizophrenia.[7]

Primary care clinics may consider recommending algorithms to primary care physicians for evaluation of dementia after a cognitive screen is positive. The American Academy of Neurology and the American Geriatrics Society have developed guidelines with recommended workup for dementia.[8] Recommended laboratory work includes testing for reversible causes of dementia, including thyroid stimulating hormone (TSH) and vitamin B12. For patients at risk of sexually transmitted infections, a rapid plasma reagin test (RPR) may be included to screen for syphilis, although it is not recommended for screening for all patients. Computed tomography or MRI brain imaging is not indicated in the evaluation of every patient with dementia, but should be considered in patients who are under the age of 60, have focal and unexplained neurologic abnormalities, have an abrupt or rapid onset over weeks to months, or who have other underlying conditions such as cancer.

When dealing with memory loss or a diagnosis of dementia, patients and caregivers may need additional support services and behavioral interventions. The Alzheimer's Association is a community-based resource that provides free support, education, and connection to community resources.[9] In many states, there is a direct referral program where physicians can directly refer patients and caregivers who have given permission to be contacted directly by the Alzheimer's Association. Studies have shown that referrals to the Alzheimer's Association from primary care lead to improved quality of dementia care, in particular, related to driving counseling, caregiver counseling, and naming of a surrogate decision maker.[10] This resource is useful for primary care physicians in supporting patients and families dealing with the challenges of caring for a patient with dementia.

Functional Assessment

Function is typically assessed by asking about ADLs and IADLs. Validated tools for functional status assessment include the Katz Activities of Daily Living (ADL) scale[11] and Lawton Instrumental Activities of Daily Living (IADL) scale.[12] See **Table 2** for examples of ADLs and IADLs. For patients who report functional limitations, the physician or clinic staff should ask additional questions about why the patient requires assistance with these tasks. Patients who now require assistance with managing finances may have transportation issues with getting to the bank, cognitive impairment leading to unpaid bills, vision loss making it difficult to balance a bank account, or hand arthritis limiting the ability to write a check. Identifying the underlying problem is important to determine how to best provide support and recommendations to improve function or to delay further functional decline. In addition, this provides an opportunity for practices to connect patients to case management or social work, or to community-based resources as needed.

Fall Risk Screening

Falls are associated with injury, hospitalization, and decreased quality of life. In addition, approximately 33% of older adults experience functional decline after a fall.[13] Fall risk screening is a required component of the initial AWV and an important step to identify opportunities to reduce the risk of future falls and functional decline for older adults.

Practice workflow redesign targeted at fall risk screening has been shown to improve both screening rates and the quality of the evaluations of patients determined to be at risk of falling.[14,15] CMS does not recommend specific questions for fall risk screening. The Assessing Care of Vulnerable Elderly interventions used the following 2 questions to assess for risk of falling:

- Have you fallen 2 or more times in the past year? Have you fallen and hurt yourself since your last doctor visit?
- Are you afraid that you might fall because of balance or walking problems?

For patients who answer "yes" to the fall risk questions in the HRA, additional evaluation should be done to evaluate for fall risk. Clinic staff can be trained to assist by checking orthostatic vital signs and by performing a structured gait assessment tool. Other approaches may include medication review, referral for a home exercise program, evaluation for an assistive device, and education of patients and families about home safety.[16] The Centers for Disease Control and Prevention has created an STEADI falls prevention toolkit that can assist providers with a multifactorial approach to preventing future falls.[17]

Depression Screening

Depression screening is a required element of the initial AWV. Although it is not required in the subsequent AWV, practices may elect to continue depression screening based on best practice recommendations. The US Preventive Services Task Force (USPSTF) recommends depression screening for adults in primary care practices "with adequate systems in place to ensure accurate diagnosis, effective treatment, and appropriate follow-up" (grade B recommendation).[18]

Validated screening tools for depression screening of older adults in primary care include the Patient Health Questionnaire 2 (PHQ-2), Patient Health Questionnaire 9, and the Geriatric Depression Scale.[19–21] The PHQ-2 is the most efficient initial screening test in primary care, involving only 2 questions, although it is not sufficient for diagnosing depression. One study has shown that increased depression screening may result in an increase in inappropriate prescribing of antidepressant medications for older adults.[22] It is important for physicians to follow-up a positive screen with a more thorough evaluation for depression and, if treatment is needed, consideration of whether medication, therapy, or social support is the most appropriate therapy for an individual patient.

An evaluation of depression screening within the AWV found that practices were not necessarily increasing the rates of depression screening along with the AWV,[23] which suggests that it is important to include depression screening in the workflow of the practice, and potentially to ensure that physicians and teams are prepared to manage positive screens for depression.

Preventive Health Care

As a preventive health benefit, the AWV is an opportunity to review a patient's preventive health care and to make recommendations about vaccinations, cancer screening, osteoporosis management, and other preventive health needs.

In older adults, preventive health recommendations have often been made based on age, although two 75 year olds may have very different prognoses. For this reason, it may be helpful to physicians to estimate a patient's life expectancy or prognosis to assist in making recommendations about preventive health care.[24] Prognosis estimates can be helpful in making recommendations about preventive health screening as well as target goals for management of conditions such as diabetes or hypertension. For instance, cancer screening with tests such as mammogram and colonoscopy is typically only recommended for patients with a life expectancy of 10 years or greater, based on the time to benefit of the screening test, so should not be recommended in patients with a shorter life expectancy, even if the patient is within the age guidelines.[25] In contrast, blood pressure control has been shown to have a time to benefit of approximately 1.5 years to reduce the risk of heart attack or stroke, so may be appropriate for patients with life expectancies of several years.[26]

Advance Directive Documentation

Studies have shown that many older adults do not have advance directives documented in their medical record. In one study of hospitalized older adults with a life expectancy of 6 months or less, only 48% of older adults had documented their health care preferences; 73% had named a health care agent, and only 30% had discussed wishes with a primary care physician.[27] Although the wishes of a patient may change over time or when facing new health care crises, advance care planning documentation has been shown to improve quality of life for older adults at the end of life, including fewer in-hospital deaths and an increased rate of referral to hospice care.[28] Interventions are needed to improve patient and decision-maker communication regarding end-of-life goals, and to increase rates of documentation of a patient's goals and wishes in the medical record. Increased rates of advance directive documentation have been demonstrated in clinics that focus on adapting clinic workflows to increase the rates of advance directives.[29]

STRATEGIES FOR INCORPORATING THE ANNUAL WELLNESS VISIT INTO CLINIC

The regulations from CMS state that the AWV may be completed by a physician (MD or DO), nonphysician practitioner (physician's assistant, nurse practitioner, or clinical nurse specialist), medical professional (including a health educator, registered dietitian, nutrition professional, or other licensed practitioner) under the supervision of a physician, or team of medical professionals who are under the direct supervision of a physician.[30] This has led to several approaches to incorporate the AWV into a busy clinic aside from having the primary clinician (ie, physician or nurse practitioner) conduct the visit.

Pharmacist-Led Visit

There are several published reports describing successful pharmacist-led AWV clinics embedded in private as well as academic primary care practices.[31–33] In many of the practices studied, the pharmacist had a one-half day or a full-day session dedicated to completing the AWV. Each practice created a list of screening tools to be used and standing orders for referrals and interventions to be placed based on the HRA and screening findings. Many reported an additional benefit of having the pharmacist review the medication list, because he or she was well equipped to identify inappropriate medications and could make adjustments as necessary. At one site, this model was associated with high patient and physician satisfaction.[33]

One large academic practice published a financial review of the feasibility of this model[34] and reported that a pharmacist who does only AWV (10% initial and 90% subsequent) would need to have an average of 2.9 visits per half day (1070 visits annually) to make it financially feasible. Of note, all of these models were in states where pharmacists have advanced clinical practitioner privileges.

Nurse-Led Visit

One health system in Topeka, Kansas[35] reported a nurse-led AWV model. In this model, a nurse saw the patient 4 to 6 weeks before seeing his or her physician, with the intention of having recommended screening tests completed in the interim so results were ready for review at the next appointment. The investigators reported a significant increase in adherences to mammogram completion but no significant difference in colonoscopy completion.

Shared Appointment

Shared appointments are group-based appointments of 6 to 12 patients, which usually last around 90 minutes. The discussion and examination can be done in the group setting. One medical group reported that they used a large conference room to hold shared AWV.[36] In this model, patients arrive with complete HRA forms, undergo hearing screening, and review paperwork with a medical behaviorist. A nurse completes vitals and vaccines, and a medical assistant identifies positive screens from the collected paperwork. The physician then reviews a presentation of USPSTF guidelines and reviews topics that are pertinent to each patient. There is a short discussion including the behaviorist, and the patient completes a checkout process.

Interprofessional Team Visit

Two teaching clinics have reported on including health professional trainees such as medical, pharmacy, and nursing students to complete the AWV while teaching learners about interprofessional care.[37,38] One family medicine clinic reported that under this model there were significant improvements in pneumococcal vaccination, mammography screen, fecal occult blood testing, and bone mineral density scanning.[37] Another clinic reported that there were mixed results about the teaching benefit of this model.[38]

SUMMARY

In summary, the AWV is an annual preventive health benefit for patients covered under Medicare to receive preventive health screening and evaluation for various geriatric syndromes. There are a variety of approaches to incorporate this visit into a busy clinic, and an opportunity for screening and evaluation of important issues in the care of older adults. Additional studies are needed to evaluate the impact of the AWV on health outcomes for older adults.

REFERENCES

1. Ganguli I, Souza J, McWilliams JM, et al. Trends in use of the US Medicare Annual Wellness Visit, 2011-2014. JAMA 2017;317(21):1–3.
2. Centers for Medicare and Medicaid Services. The ABCs of the Annual Wellness Visit (AWV). Available at: https://www.cms.gov/Outreach-and-Education/Medicare-Learning-Network-MLN/MLNProducts/downloads/AWV_chart_ICN905706.pdf. Accessed June 12, 2017.
3. Centers for Medicare and Medicaid Services. Frequently asked questions from the March 28, 2012 Medicare Preventive Services national provider call: the initial preventive physical exam and the Annual Wellness Visit. Available at: https://www.cms.gov/Outreach-and-Education/Outreach/NPC/Downloads/IPPE-AWV-FAQs.pdf. Accessed June 12, 2017.
4. Bradford A, Kunik ME, Schulz P, et al. Missed and delayed diagnosis of dementia in primary care: prevalence and contributing factors. Alzheimer Dis Assoc Disord 2009;23(4):306–14.
5. Cordell CB, Borson S, Boustani M, et al. Alzheimer's Association recommendations for operationalizing the detection of cognitive impairment during the Medicare Annual Wellness Visit in a primary care setting. Alzheimers Dement 2013; 9(2):141–50.
6. Brodaty H, Low L-F, Gibson L, et al. What is the best dementia screening instrument for general practitioners to use? Am J Geriatr Psychiatry 2006;14(5): 391–400.
7. American Psychiatric Association. Diagnostic and statistical manual of mental disorders. 5th edition. Arlington (VA): American Psychiatric Association; 2013.
8. AGS Clinical Practice Committee. Guidelines abstracted from the American Academy of Neurology's Dementia guidelines for early detection, diagnosis, and management of dementia. J Am Geriatr Soc 2003;51(6):869–73.
9. Alzheimer's Association. alz.org. Available at: http://www.alz.org/. Published 2017. Accessed December 6, 2017.
10. Reuben DB, Roth CP, Frank JC, et al. Assessing care of vulnerable elders - Alzheimer's disease: a pilot study of a practice redesign intervention to improve the quality of dementia care. J Am Geriatr Soc 2010;58(2):324–9.
11. Katz S, Downs TD, Cash HR, et al. Progress in development of the index of ADL. Gerontologist 1970;10(1):20–30.
12. Lawton MP, Brody EM. Assessment of older people: self-maintaining and instrumental activities of daily living. Gerontologist 1969;9(3):179–86.
13. Covinsky KE, Palmer RM, Fortinsky RH, et al. Loss of independence in activities of daily living in older adults hospitalized with medical illnesses: increased vulnerability with age. J Am Geriatr Soc 2003;51(4):451–8.
14. Ganz DA, Kim SB, Zingmond DS, et al. Effect of a falls quality improvement program on serious fall-related injuries. J Am Geriatr Soc 2015;63(1):63–70.
15. Wenger NS, Roth CA, Hall WJ, et al. Practice redesign to improve care for falls and urinary incontinence. JAMA Intern Med 2017;170(19):1765–72.
16. Gillespie LD, Robertson MC, Gillespie WJ, et al. Interventions for preventing falls in older people living in the community. Cochrane Database Syst Rev 2009;(2):CD007146.
17. Stevens JA, Phelan EA. Development of STEADI. Health Promot Pract 2013;14(5): 706–14.
18. Siu AL, Bibbins-Domingo K, Grossman DC, et al. Screening for depression in adults. JAMA 2016;315(4):380.

19. Phelan E, Williams B, Meeker K, et al. A study of the diagnostic accuracy of the PHQ-9 in primary care elderly. BMC Fam Pract 2010;11(1):63.
20. Almeida OP, Almeida SA. Short versions of the geriatric depression scale: a study of their validity for the diagnosis of a major depressive episode according to ICD-10 and DSM-IV. Int J Geriatr Psychiatry 1999;14(1):858–65.
21. Li C, Friedman B, Conwell Y, et al. Validity of the Patient Health Questionnaire 2 (PHQ-2) in identifying major depression in older people. J Am Geriatr Soc 2007;55(4):596–602.
22. Rhee TG, Capistrant BD, Schommer JC, et al. Effects of depression screening on diagnosing and treating mood disorders among older adults in office-based primary care outpatient settings: An instrumental variable analysis. Prev Med 2017; 100:101–11.
23. Pfoh E, Mojtabai R, Bailey J, et al. Impact of medicare Annual Wellness Visits on uptake of depression screening. Psychiatr Serv 2015;66(11):1207.
24. Pollack CE, Blackford AL, Schoenborn NL, et al. Comparing prognostic tools for cancer screening: considerations for clinical practice and performance assessment. J Am Geriatr Soc 2016;64(5):1032–8.
25. Lee SJ, Boscardin WJ, Stijacic-Cenzer I, et al. Time lag to benefit after screening for breast and colorectal cancer: meta-analysis of survival data from the United States, Sweden, United Kingdom, and Denmark. BMJ 2012;346:e8441.
26. Patel A, MacMahon S, Chalmers J, et al. Effects of a fixed combination of perindopril and indapamide on macrovascular and microvascular outcomes in patients with type 2 diabetes mellitus (the ADVANCE trial): a randomised controlled trial. Lancet 2007;370(9590):829–40.
27. Heyland DK, Barwich D, Pichora D, et al. Failure to engage hospitalized elderly patients and their families in advance care planning. JAMA Intern Med 2013; 173(9):778–87.
28. Bischoff KE, Sudore R, Miao Y, et al. Advance care planning and the quality of end-of-life care in older adults. J Am Geriatr Soc 2013;61(2):209–14.
29. Kamo N, Williams BL, Smith DL, et al. Improving the electronic capture of advance care directives in a healthcare delivery system. J Am Geriatr Soc 2017;65(5):973–9.
30. Centers for Medicare and Medicaid Services. Medicare benefit policy manual. In: 228th edition. CMS Pub; 2016. 280.5. Available at: https://www.cms.gov/Regulations-and-Guidance/Guidance/Manuals/Downloads/bp102c15.pdf. Accessed October 3, 2017.
31. Warshany K, Sherrill CH, Cavanaugh J, et al. Medicare Annual Wellness Visits conducted by a pharmacist in an internal medicine clinic. Am J Health Syst Pharm 2014;71(1):44–9.
32. Thomas MH, Goode JV. Development and implementation of a pharmacist-delivered Medicare Annual Wellness Visit at a family practice office. J Am Pharm Assoc 2014;54(4):427–34.
33. Wilson CG, Park I, Sutherland SE, et al. Assessing pharmacist-led Annual Wellness Visits: interventions made and patient and physician satisfaction. J Am Pharm Assoc 2015;55(4):449–54.
34. Park I, Sutherland SE, Ray L, et al. Financial implications of pharmacist-led medicare Annual Wellness Visits. J Am Pharm Assoc 2014;54(4):435–40.
35. Tetuan TM, Ohm R, Herynk MH, et al. The affordable health care act Annual Wellness Visits. J Nurs Adm 2014;44(5):270–5.
36. Kainkaryam V. The Annual Wellness Visit shared medical appointment. J Ambul Care Manage 2013;36(4):335–7.

37. Zorek JA, Subash M, Fike DS, et al. Impact of an interprofessional teaching clinic on preventive care services. Fam Med 2015;47(7):558–61.
38. Irons B, Evans L, Bogschutz R, et al. Utilising Medicare Annual Wellness Visits to implement interprofessional education in the primary care setting. J Interprof Care 2016;30(4):529–31.

Individualized Approach to Cancer Screening in Older Adults

Kimberley T. Lee, MD[a],*, Russell P. Harris, MD, MPH[b],
Nancy L. Schoenborn, MD[a]

KEYWORDS

- Cancer screening • Personalized medicine • Life expectancy • Harms and benefits
- Older adults

KEY POINTS

- Cancer screening in older adults is associated with uncertainty with a small degree of benefit that is not evident until many years later but harms that could occur immediately.
- Health status and functional status vary considerably among older adults, which leads to significant heterogeneity in benefit-risk considerations.
- Individualization of cancer screening decision involves considering the degree of benefits and harms, time horizon to benefits in relation to life expectancy, time horizon to harms, and patient preferences.

INTRODUCTION

Cancer screening increases the chance of detecting cancers early but is also associated with several potential harms.[1-4] The screening decision needs to balance the likelihood for benefit versus the likelihood for harm, consider the time horizon to benefit versus the time horizon to harm, and incorporate patient preference.[5-8] Because all of these considerations vary depending on individual level factors, a more individualized approach to cancer screening is important. An individualized approach is especially critical for older adults because of the high degree of heterogeneity in both the health status and the health trajectory among this population, which then leads to significant variation in the benefit-harm considerations related to cancer screening.[5,9]

Disclosure Statement: The authors have no financial disclosures.
[a] Department of Medicine, Johns Hopkins University School of Medicine, 5200 Eastern Avenue, Mason F Lord Building Center Tower, Room 711, Baltimore, MD 21224, USA; [b] Division of General Medicine and Clinical Epidemiology, Sheps Center for Health Services Research, University of North Carolina, 101 Parkview Crescent, Chapel Hill, NC 27516, USA
* Corresponding author. 1650 Orleans Street, CRB1 186, Baltimore, MD 21287.
E-mail address: klee149@jhmi.edu

In this article, the authors review key considerations in a more individualized approach to screening; they review current guidelines regarding cancer screening in older adults and propose frameworks in the literature that are relevant to individualized cancer screening. Finally, they discuss tools and challenges to implementing an individualized approach for cancer screening. Discussions focus around breast, colorectal, and prostate cancer screening as examples, because these are the most common cancer screenings in older adults. The objectives are to provide an overview of how to better tailor the cancer screening decision so that benefits outweigh the harms and to acknowledge the gaps and limitations in the available evidence that need to be addressed as next steps.

WHAT TO CONSIDER IN AN INDIVIDUALIZED APPROACH TO CANCER SCREENING
Magnitude of Benefit and Time Horizon to Benefit

One's potential benefit from cancer screening depends on 3 factors: (1) the baseline risk for a specific type of cancer in the absence of screening; (2) the relative risk reduction from screening; and (3) the time horizon over which the risk reduction occurs. Each of these factors is discussed later.

One common and practical consideration when thinking about baseline risk for cancer is to categorize patients as above average risk (have known risk factors for developing a certain type of cancer) or average risk (have no known risk factors). Many risk factors can be easily assessed in routine care of older adults (**Table 1**).[2–4,10–12] Guidelines on cancer screening and studies on the benefits of cancer screening focus on those at average risk.[2–4] Less data are available to guide the management of those with above average risk. Patients who have genetic predispositions for higher risks of certain cancers, such as BRCA gene mutations for breast and ovarian cancers, or familial adenomatous polyposis for colorectal cancer (CRC), should be considered separately (use available guidelines specific to the risk factor) and referrals to specialists such as high risk cancer screening clinics are reasonable[10–12]; however, it is unlikely that these issues are first discovered in older adults. The nongenetic cancer risk factors are often epidemiologic associations without clear causal link.[13] Although it is intuitive to think that patients with these risk factors would stand to benefit more from screening, and a more aggressive screening approach may be reasonable, it is important to note that there is uncertainty about whether screening is more beneficial in this population. This is because screening is beneficial only for certain subtypes of

Table 1 Risk factors for breast, colorectal, and prostate cancers			
	Breast Cancer	**Colorectal Cancer**	**Prostate Cancer**
Risk factors	• Age • Family history • Race/ethnicity • BRCA 1 or BRCA 2 gene • Time of first menstrual period • Time of first birth of child	• Age • Family history • Race/ethnicity • Inflammatory bowel disease • Familial adenomatous polyposis • Body mass index • Vegetable intake • Use of NSAIDs • Smoking history	• Age • Family history • Race/ethnicity • Urinary symptoms

Data from Refs.[2–4,10–12]

cancer; screening is not beneficial, for example, regarding those cancers that are slow-growing and would never become clinically relevant or those cancer that are extremely aggressive and can develop in between screenings.[3,5,7,8] More studies are needed to better quantify the degree of risk reduction offered by screening among individuals who are at above average risk to develop specific cancers.

The benefit of screening is commonly represented by reduction in cancer-specific mortality. The authors focus on absolute risk reduction, which is more clinically meaningful. For breast cancer screening, repeat screening mammography between the ages of 50 and 74 reduces 7 breast cancer deaths per 1000 screened over a lifetime, or an absolute risk reduction of 0.7%.[13] For CRC screening, regular screening between the ages of 50 and 75 is estimated to reduce CRC death by 17 to 24 per 1000 screening over a lifetime, or an absolute risk reduction of 1.7% to 2.4%.[14] For prostate cancer screening, the benefit of screening remains controversial. An update to the US Preventive Services Task Force (USPSTF) recommendation mentions that screening in men between the ages of 55 and 69 showed reduction of prostate cancer death only in 1 study, by 1 to 2 per 1000 screened or absolute risk reduction of 0.1% to 0.2%.[15,16] An often underemphasized aspect of these data is that these estimates are based on *repeated* screening over a 15- to 25-year time period; the risk reduction from each individual screening test is likely significantly smaller.

Not only are the benefit estimates based on repeated screening over long time periods, but also these benefits do not become apparent until a much delayed time point from the time of initial screening. The absolute risk reduction cited above is over the course of *lifetime*, and a recent meta-analysis has shown that the time horizon to achieve one saved life from screening out of every 1000 persons screened is 9 to 10 years for breast and CRCs.[17] For prostate cancer, controversies remain whether screening provides any mortality benefit, but one study that suggested mortality benefit had a lag-time to benefit of around 13 years.[15] This becomes significant for those older adults who have limited life expectancy and may not live long enough to benefit.[2–4] A related concept is that of competing risks: more than half of all older adults have multiple chronic conditions and some may be more likely to die with an indolent cancer from other illnesses than from that cancer.[18,19] Consider a 65-year-old man with stage 4 chronic kidney disease, poorly controlled hypertension, and end-stage heart failure; this person's estimated life expectancy is less than 5 years. Even if colonic polyps were present, this person is far more likely to die of his other serious illnesses before the polyps progress to be clinically relevant. The diagnosis of cancers that would otherwise not have become a threat to health, or even apparent, during one's lifetime is known as overdiagnosis. Approximately 30% of all screening-detected breast cancers and up to 50% of screening-detected prostate cancers may be overdiagnosis, which are usually 3 to 4 times the number of lives that are saved by screening.[13,16,20,21] Overdiagnosis can cause substantial psychological and emotional distress and also lead to overtreatment that is associated with significant harms and burdens.[20–22]

In light of cancer screening's long lag-time to benefit and the multiple competing risks for mortality in older adults, a patient's life expectancy should be considered. Compared with younger populations, older adults are much more heterogeneous in their health status and health trajectories. For example, adults at age 80 can have life expectancies that range from months to more than 10 years.[9]

Potential Harms and Burdens of Screening

The potential harms from screening tests are numerous. In contrast to the delayed benefit from screening, these harms almost all occur immediately after screening and many can have long-lasting effects.[2-4] More obvious harms include the direct complications from screening tests, such as perforation, bleeding, and anesthesia reactions from colonoscopy, radiation exposure, and discomfort from mammography.[23] Other harms include false positives and the complications from downstream diagnostic testing, such as pain and infection risks from prostate and breast biopsies, and overdiagnosis and overtreatment of clinically unimportant cancers.[5,6] Less often considered are the psychological stress from screening, burden of the screening and downstream testing to patients, and diverted attention away from other health conditions or more impactful health interventions.[6,7,24] Clinicians often have limited time during clinic visits; time spent discussing cancer screening diverts time that could be spent on counseling on other health issues that may be significantly more beneficial for older adults.[25]

The risks for many of these harms increase with age. Using screening colonoscopy as an example, older adults aged 80 to 84 have almost 80% increased risk of serious gastrointestinal events such as perforation or gastrointestinal bleeding, or requiring blood transfusions compared with those aged 66 to 69 (8.8 vs 5.0 events per 1000 procedures).[23] The risk of other gastrointestinal events, such as ileus, nausea, emesis, and dehydration, are more than doubled for older adults (15.9 vs 6.9 events per 1000). The risks for harms also increase with comorbidities. For instance, risk of serious gastrointestinal events more than doubles for those with stroke or heart failure and increases by 50% for those with chronic obstructive pulmonary disease.[23] Furthermore, older adults are more likely to have sensory or cognitive deficits that make screening tests more burdensome or frightening.[5] In this context, assessment of the risks for these potential harms for each individual patient is essential among older adults with multiple chronic conditions.

Informed Patient Preference

Patient preference is important to screening decision for several reasons. First, the application of population-based data to an individual involves inherent uncertainties and assumptions. One cannot predict the exact cancer risk or the exact life expectancy of any individual. Rather, there is evidence on probabilities of various events. As such, patients may have different thresholds for what is an acceptable benefit/harm ratio for screening. For example, a woman with a family history of a cousin with breast cancer does not rise to the level of increased risk of breast cancer for that patient. However, she may have a strong preference for screening due to a higher level of fear for cancer and is willing to accept a higher risk for harm relative to benefit from screening. Second, a patient may value outcomes other than reduced mortality and morbidity related to cancer. For example, some patients value the sense of reassurance or the knowledge of whether they have cancer, even if they may not desire treatment.[26]

Eliciting patient preference may be often challenging. Patients commonly overestimate the benefits of screening while underestimating the harms.[27,28] Other patients may misunderstand the purpose of screening and perceive the need for testing to be linked with presence of symptoms.[29] In these instances, helping patients to adequately understand the benefits and harms associated with screening is crucial before eliciting preference; this can be a time-consuming and demanding task, especially for those patients with limited health literacy and numeracy. Furthermore, preferences are susceptible to the context and framing of the information. For example, messaging in terms of "survival" is more influential on decision making than messaging in terms of "mortality."[30] Patients also have different preferred decision-making roles; sometimes, a person's preference is for the clinician to make the decision.[31] Ongoing research is actively investigating optimal communication strategies and tools to facilitate the discussion of screening in a more individualized approach. In the meantime, one way to move forward may be to first understand any strong opinions the patient has toward screening and the basis for those opinions, to then provide a recommendation based on available evidence on benefits and harms, and provide more details if the patient disagrees with the recommendation or desires additional information.

WHAT DO THE GUIDELINES SAY REGARDING INDIVIDUALIZED CANCER SCREENING?

The guidelines for breast, colorectal, and prostate cancer screening put forth by the USPSTF, the American Cancer Society (ACS), the American College of Physicians (ACP), and the National Comprehensive Cancer Network (NCCN) are briefly reviewed, with a focus on recommendations relevant to an individualized approach to cancer screening in older adults (**Table 2**).[1,10–12,14,16,32–36] Most of the recommendations around individualized decision making involve situations where the benefits and harms of screening are more uncertain or evidence is lacking; as such, these are also the situations where the guidelines from different societies are at times inconsistent.

Breast Cancer Screening

All guidelines referenced recommend screening mammography as the test of choice for breast cancer screening.[1,12,13,33] One area for individualized decision making is the frequency of screening mammography. The USPSTF and the ACP recommend biennial screening mammography for women aged 50 to 74.[1,13] The NCCN recommends annual screening for women over the age of 40.[12] The ACS recommends annual mammograms for women 45 to 54 years old and biennial mammograms for women 55 years and older (although they can make individualized decision to continue annual screening).[33] The authors propose using biennial screening as the default to minimize the potential harm of false positives, which increases with frequency of screening, because there is no evidence that annual screening provides additional benefit in those 50 to 74.

A second area for individualization is the time to stop screening. The USPSTF has found insufficient evidence to make a recommendation for women older than 74 years of age.[13] The NCCN recommends an individualized decision for women over the age of 65, "weighing its potential benefits/risks in the context of the patients overall health and estimated longevity."[12] They also recommend against screening if a patient cannot undergo treatment due to comorbidities or is not expected to live long enough to benefit from screening (<10 years) regardless of age.[12] The ACS recommends that screening should continue as long as life expectancy exceeds 10 years and to take into account patient preferences when making breast cancer screening decision for older women with life expectancy of at least 10 years.[33] The ACP recommends against screening women older than 75 years of age or if life expectancy is less than 10 years.[1]

Colorectal Cancer Screening

Screening tests recommended for colorectal screening include colonoscopy every 10 years, high-sensitivity fecal occult blood test or fecal immunochemical test annually, and sigmoidoscopy every 5 years.[10,14,34,35] The choice of screening test modality is to be individualized based on patient preference and local availability.

Regarding the age to stop screening, both the USPSTF and the NCCN recommend CRC screening for adults aged 50 to 75.[10,14] They recommend an individualized

Table 2
Summary of screening recommendations from US Preventive Services Task Force, National Comprehensive Cancer Network, American Cancer Society, and American College of Physicians

A. Breast Cancer

	Test of Choice	Screening Interval	When to Begin, y	When to Stop
USPSTF	Mammography	Biennial	50	75 y
NCCN	Mammography	Annual	40	If cannot tolerate treatment or will not live long enough to benefit
ACS	Mammogram	Annual Biennial	45 55	Poor health and life expectancy <10 y
ACP	Mammography	Biennial	50	75 y or older or life expectancy <10 y

B. Colorectal Cancer

	Test of Choice with Screening Interval	When to Begin, y	When to Stop
USPSTF	Annual guaiac-based fecal occult blood test (g-FOBT) Annual FIT, FIT DNA annually or every 3 y, colonoscopy every 10 y, CT colonography every 5 y, flexible sigmoidoscopy every 5 y, flexible sigmoidoscopy every 10 y plus annual FIT	50	76 y
NCCN	Colonoscopy every 10 y, gFOBT or FIT annually, DNA-based testing every 3 y, flexible sigmoidoscopy every 5 y ± FIT at year 3, CT colonography every 5 y	50	76 y
ACS	Colonoscopy every 10 y, flexible sigmoidoscopy every 5 y, double-contrast barium enema every 5 y, CT colonography every 5 y	50	Not specified
ACP	Annual gFOBT or FIT, flexible sigmoidoscopy every 5 y, colonoscopy every 10 y	50	76 y or life expectancy <10 y

C. Prostate Cancer

	Test of Choice	When to Begin	When to Stop
USPSTF	Recommends against PSA-based screening	N/A	N/A
NCCN	PSA (interval determined by PSA result)	45 y	75 y or >60 y with PSA <1
ACS	PSA ± DRE (interval determined by PSA result)	50 y (individualized decision)	Not specified
ACP	PSA	50 y (individualized decision)	76 y or life expectancy <10 y

Abbreviations: CT, computed tomography; DRE, digital rectal examination; FIT, fecal immunochemical test.

Data from (A) Refs.[1,12,13,33]; (B) Refs.[10,14,34,35]; and (C) Refs.[11,16,32,36]

decision be made for adult aged 76 to 85 years. The USPSTF adds that patients who can tolerate treatment and do not have reduced life expectancy are also more likely to benefit.[14] The ACS recommends that CRC screening begin at age 50, but does not specify reasons to stop screening.[34] The ACP recommends screening for adults aged 50 to 74 and recommends against screening patients older than 75 years of age or if life expectancy is less than 10 years.[35]

Prostate Cancer Screening

Prostate cancer screening is a controversial topic. The current USPSTF recommendation is against prostate-specific antigen (PSA) testing for prostate cancer screening for all ages, although in the draft update, it proposes an individualized decision be made for those 55 to 69.[16] The NCCN recommends an individualized decision based on discussion of risks and benefits of screening.[11] For men older than 75 years, they state that testing "should be done with caution and only in very healthy men with little or no comorbidity" given the risk of overdiagnosis. The NCCN guidelines also state that men over the age of 60 with PSA less than 1 ng/mL are not likely to benefit from further screening. The ACS recommends individualized decision for men 45 and older but against screening men with life expectancy less than 10 years.[32] The ACP recommends an individualized decision for men aged 50 to 69 using risk of prostate cancer, risks and benefits of screening, health status and life expectancy as well as patient preferences, but they recommend against screening men outside of that age range and men with life expectancy less than 10 to 15 years.[36]

Common Theme

One common theme in the recommendations that mention individualized decision making is using the patient's age, health status, and life expectancy to inform when to stop screening or, in the case of prostate cancer, whether to screen at all.[1,10–14,16,32–36] It may be helpful to recall that the implicit basis for these considerations is the more fundamental, weighing of the likelihood of benefits against the likelihood for harms. As discussed previously, the probability of harms increases with age and with comorbidities. Therefore, even in those older adults who are likely to live long enough to have a reasonable probability of benefitting from screening, the balance between benefits and harms is usually different than that of younger adults, and thoughtful balance of the 2 is crucial.

TOOLS THAT FACILITATE INDIVIDUALIZED APPROACH TO CANCER SCREENING
Tools to Estimate Risk of Cancer

Multiple models are available to predict risk of development of cancer in adults. There are at least 17 models for breast cancer, 127 for prostate cancer, and 9 for CRC.[37] Some of the more accessible tools are presented in later discussion.

One breast cancer risk assessment tool, available at https://www.cancer.gov/bcrisktool/, compares an individual woman's risk of developing breast cancer in 5 years to a woman of the same age with average risk factors for women aged 35 to 85. It also provides an estimate of the lifetime risk of developing breast cancer. The tool takes into consideration personal history of breast cancer, ductal carcinoma in situ, or lobular carcinoma in situ, BRCA mutation, age, age of menarche, age of first live birth, first-degree relatives with breast cancer, history of biopsy, and race.

The National Cancer Institute has developed a CRC risk assessment tool (https://www.cancer.gov/colorectalcancerrisk/). The model is directed at adults 50 to 85 years old.[38,39] It a takes into account age, ethnicity, body mass index, vegetable intake, history of polyps, use of nonsteroidal anti-inflammatory drugs (NSAIDs), exercise, smoking history, family history, and estrogen status for women and provides 5-year, 10-year, and lifetime estimates of risk of developing CRC compared with average.

Several models predict prostate cancer risk but require results from PSA testing, digital rectal examination, or genetic markers.[15,40–42] One model that can be used without PSA testing is the European Randomized study of Screening for Prostate Cancer (ERSPC) risk calculator (http://www.prostatecancer-riskcalculator.com/), which calculates the risk of prostate cancer compared with average based on age, family history, and urinary symptoms assessed by the American Urological Association symptom score.[15,43] For men who elect to have PSA done, the ERSPC calculator can further stratify risk of prostate cancer and guide decisions about additional workups.

Tools to Estimate Life Expectancy

Incorporating life expectancy to inform individualized cancer screening decisions is endorsed by multiple professional societies. Several models that estimate long-term life expectancy over 9 to 10 years among community-dwelling older adults demonstrate good calibration and discrimination; these models use commonly available information, including age, comorbidities, and functional status and can be found at www.eprognosis.org.[44,45] Gait speed has also been shown to be predictive of life expectancy with gait speed of 0.8 m/s associated with median life expectancy, while faster and slower gait speeds are associated with longer and shorter life expectancies, respectively.[46] Although it is not a commonly performed assessment in primary care, it requires little training or equipment for it to become more widely used. The Charlson Comorbidity Index (CCI) uses a scale of weighted comorbidity to estimate mortality (Excel macro tool available).[47,48] A CCI score of 0, 1 to 2, 3 to 4, or greater than 5 carries a 1-year risk of mortality of 12%, 26%, 52%, and 85% mortality, respectively.

Frameworks for Individualizing Cancer Screening Decisions

The most well-known framework was developed by Walter and Covinsky[5] and considers risk of dying from screen-detectable cancer, the benefit of cancer screening, the harms of screening, and using patient values and preferences to anchor the final decision. The investigators use estimated life expectancy and age-specific cancer mortalities to estimate the risk of dying from a specific type of cancer in the remaining lifetime of a given patient, and conversely, the number needed to screen to prevent 1 cancer-specific death. This framework of using remainder lifetime as the metric for risk presentation is easily understandable; it also carries the benefit of presenting a lower cancer-specific lifetime risk for the older, sicker patients (due to competing risks), which can be more palatable for patients to accept.

Subsequent work by Lee and colleagues[17] proposes to compare a person's predicted life expectancy to the lag-time to benefit from screening. If life expectancy is significantly longer than lag-time to benefit, then screening should be recommended. If the converse is true, then screening should stop. If life expectancy and lag-time to benefit are comparable, then patient preference should drive the decision. This framework emphasizes the important consideration of the long lag-time to benefit from screening but does not account for comparison of the magnitude of benefit to the potential harms. In addition, the lag-time to benefit depends on the threshold for risk reduction. For example, to achieve 1 averted cancer death out of 1000 screened for CRC, the lag-time to this degree of benefit is approximately 10 years, but if a threshold of 2 averted cancer deaths out of 1000 is chosen, then the lag-time to benefit is closer to 15 years.[49]

Harris and colleagues[50] proposed a value-based framework that considers not only the benefits and harms of screening but also the costs and intensity of screening

(**Fig. 1**). Screening intensity is defined to incorporate the population that is screened (for example, screening in older adults with limited life expectancy is considered high intensity screening), frequency of screening, and sensitivity of tests. The framework posits that low-value care can result from either low benefits or high harms and costs. Low-intensity strategies are initially low-value because of low benefit. As intensity increases, benefits increase and value increases until benefits are outweighed by harms and costs, at which point the high-end extreme of screening intensity again leads to low-value care.

CHALLENGES AROUND INDIVIDUALIZED CANCER SCREENING

Several knowledge gaps exist. Older adults are frequently underrepresented in clinical trials of cancer screening.[51] There is currently no available model that synthesizes the predicted risk for cancer with the predicted life expectancy. For example, for someone with above average risk for cancer but also a limited life expectancy, there is no guidance on how to balance those 2 estimates to reach an evidence-based decision. There is also no consensus on whether evidence or patient demand should dictate the final cancer screening decision.

Other challenges to implementing individualized approach to cancer screening include health care system and communication barriers. Health care organizations that measure quality of care based on screening rate in a specific age group may potentially penalize clinicians if an individualized approach led to different decisions than suggested by the guidelines. In one study, screening rate of health 76-year-old men was much lower than that of sick 75-year-old men because of the quality indicator set at age 75 or younger.[52] Another system barrier is the excessive public enthusiasm toward cancer screening. In one national survey study of 500 adults over the age of 40 years, 87% of respondents believed that routine cancer screening is usually a good idea, 66% wanted to be screened for cancer even if it could not be treated, and 41% thought that an 80-year-old choosing to forego cancer screening is irresponsible.[53] There is a need for improving public's education about the risks of cancer screening to help facilitate more balanced decisions.

Clinicians may struggle with how to discuss stopping screening because of concerns about patient expectations or discomfort with communicating life

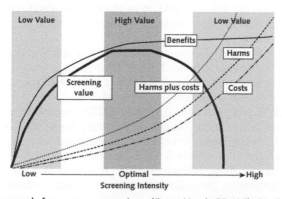

Fig. 1. Value framework for cancer screening. (*From* Harris RP, Wilt TJ, Qaseem A, et al. A value framework for cancer screening: advice for high-value care from the American College of Physicians. Ann Intern Med 2015;162(10):712; with permission.)

expectancy.[54–56] One small study showed, encouragingly, that older adults were open to screening cessation and did not have negative reactions to such a recommendation from the clinicians.[29]

SUMMARY

A thoughtful balance of the probability, magnitude, and the relevant time horizon of benefit and of harm is needed in making screening recommendations for older adults. It is realized that such an approach can be significantly more complex and time-intensive than using simple age thresholds and that it is still a work in progress as more data are being gathered to address the knowledge gaps and barriers described above. It is nonetheless critically important because the goal of cancer screening, as with all other medical care, is first to do no harm. This article highlights that, as age and comorbidities increase, the benefit of screening becomes more uncertain while the probability for harms from screening becomes higher. The recognition of this evidence is a first step toward a more individualized approach to cancer screening in older adults.

REFERENCES

1. Wilt TJ, Harris RP, Qaseem A, High Value Care Task Force of the American College of Physicians. Screening for cancer: advice for high-value care from the American College of Physicians. Ann Intern Med 2015;162(10):718–25.
2. Lin JS, Piper MA, Perdue LA, et al. Screening for colorectal cancer: updated evidence report and systematic review for the US Preventive Services Task Force. JAMA 2016;315(23):2576–94.
3. Nelson HD, Fu R, Cantor A, et al. Effectiveness of breast cancer screening: systematic review and meta-analysis to update the 2009 U.S. Preventive Services Task Force recommendation. Ann Intern Med 2016;164(4):244–55.
4. Ilic D, Neuberger MM, Djulbegovic M, et al. Screening for prostate cancer. Cochrane Database Syst Rev 2013;(1):CD004720.
5. Walter LC, Covinsky KE. Cancer screening in elderly patients: a framework for individualized decision making. JAMA 2001;285(21):2750–6.
6. Lansdorp-Vogelaar I, Gulati R, Mariotto AB, et al. Personalizing age of cancer screening cessation based on comorbidity: model estimates of harms and benefits. Ann Intern Med 2014;161(2):104–12.
7. Breslau ES, Gorin SS, Edwards HM, et al. An individualized approach to cancer screening decisions in older adults: a multilevel framework. J Gen Intern Med 2016;31(5):539–47.
8. Soung MC. Screening for cancer: when to stop?: a practical guide and review of the evidence. Med Clin North Am 2015;99(2):249–62.
9. Reuben DB. Medical care for the final years of life: "When you're 83, it's not going to be 20 years". JAMA 2009;302(24):2686–94.
10. Provenzale D, Gupta S, Ahnen DJ, et al. NCCN guidelines colorectal cancer screening version 2.2016. Available at: https://www.nccn.org/professionals/physician_gls/pdf/colorectal_screening.pdf. Accessed May 18, 2017.
11. Carroll PR, Parsons JK, Andriole G, et al. NCCN Guidelines prostate cancer early detection version 2.2016. Published 2016. Available at: https://www.nccn.org/professionals/physician_gls/pdf/prostate_detection.pdf. Accessed May 18, 2017.
12. Bevers TB, Helvie M, Bonaccio E, et al. NCCN guidelines. Breast cancer screening and diagnosis (version 2.2016). Published 2016. Available at: https://

www.nccn.org/professionals/physician_gls/pdf/breast-screening.pdf. Accessed May 18, 2017.

13. Siu AL, U.S. Preventive Services Task Force. Screening for breast cancer: U.S. Preventive Services Task Force recommendation statement. Ann Intern Med 2016;164(4):279–96.

14. Bibbins-Domingo K, Grossman DC, Curry SJ, et al. Screening for colorectal cancer: U.S. Preventive Services Task Force Recommendation Statement. JAMA 2016;315(23):2564–75.

15. Roobol MJ, Steyerberg EW, Kranse R, et al. A risk-based strategy improves prostate-specific antigen–driven detection of prostate cancer. Eur Urol 2010; 57(1):79–85.

16. Moyer VA, U.S. Preventive Services Task Force. Screening for prostate cancer: U.S. Preventive Services Task force recommendation statement. Ann Intern Med 2012;157(2):120–34.

17. Lee SJ, Leipzig RM, Walter LC. Incorporating lag time to benefit into prevention decisions for older adults. JAMA 2013;310(24):2609–10.

18. Gerteis J, Izrael D, Deitz D, et al. Multiple chronic conditions chartbook. AHRQ Publ No, Q13-0038. 2014:52. Available at: http://www.ahrq.gov/professionals/prevention-chronic-care/decision/mcc/mccchartbook.pdf. Accessed May 18, 2017.

19. Guiding principles for the care of older adults with multimorbidity: an approach for clinicians. Guiding principles for the care of older adults with multimorbidity: an approach for clinicians: American Geriatrics Society Expert Panel on the care of older adults with multimorbidity. J Am Geriatr Soc 2012;60(10):E1–25.

20. Bleyer A, Welch HG. Effect of three decades of screening mammography on breast-cancer incidence. N Engl J Med 2012;367(21):1998–2005.

21. Baum M. Harms from breast cancer screening outweigh benefits if death caused by treatment is included. BMJ 2013;346:f385.

22. Harris JV. Ductal carcinoma in situ stage 0 breast cancer. JAMA Intern Med 2016; 176(7):887.

23. Warren JL, Klabunde CN, Mariotto AB, et al. Adverse events after outpatient colonoscopy in the Medicare population. Ann Intern Med 2009;150(12):849–57.

24. Lerman C, Trock B, Rimer BK, et al. Psychological side effects of breast cancer screening. Health Psychol 1991;10(4):259–67.

25. Eckstrom E, Feeny DH, Walter LC, et al. Individualizing cancer screening in older adults: a narrative review and framework for future research. J Gen Intern Med 2013;28(2):292–8.

26. Schonberg MA, McCarthy EP, York M, et al. Factors influencing elderly women's mammography screening decisions: implications for counseling. BMC Geriatr 2007;7(1):26.

27. Sutkowi-Hemstreet A, Vu M, Harris R, et al. Adult patients' perspectives on the benefits and harms of overused screening tests: a qualitative study. J Gen Intern Med 2015;30(11):1618–26.

28. Hoffman RM, Lewis CL, Pignone MP, et al. Decision-making processes for breast, colorectal, and prostate cancer screening: the DECISIONS survey. Med Decis Making 2010;30(5 Suppl):53S–64S.

29. Schoenborn NL, Lee KT, Pollack CE, et al. Older adults' views and communication preferences about cancer screening cessation. JAMA Intern Med 2017; 177(8):1121–8.

30. Veldwijk J, Essers BAB, Lambooij MS, et al. Survival or mortality: does risk attribute framing influence decision-making behavior in a discrete choice experiment? Value Health 2016;19(2):202–9.
31. Degner LF, Kristjanson LJ, Bowman D, et al. Information needs and decisional preferences in women with breast cancer. JAMA 1997;277(18):1485–92.
32. Wolf AMD, Wender RC, Etzioni RB, et al. American Cancer Society Guideline for the early detection of prostate cancer: update 2010. CA Cancer J Clin 2010; 60(2):70–98.
33. Oeffinger KC, Fontham ETH, Etzioni R, et al. Breast cancer screening for women at average risk. JAMA 2015;314(15):1599–614.
34. Levin B, Lieberman DA, McFarland B, et al. Screening and surveillance for the early detection of colorectal cancer and adenomatous polyps, 2008: a joint guideline from the American Cancer Society, the US Multi-Society Task Force on colorectal cancer, and the American College of Radiology. CA Cancer J Clin 2008;58(3):130–60.
35. Qaseem A, Denberg TD, Hopkins RH, et al. Screening for colorectal cancer: a guidance statement from the American College of Physicians. Ann Intern Med 2012;156(5):378–86.
36. Qaseem A, Barry MJ, Denberg TD, et al, Clinical Guidelines Committee of the American College of Physicians. Screening for prostate cancer: a guidance statement from the Clinical Guidelines Committee of the American College of Physicians. Ann Intern Med 2013;158(10):761–9.
37. Usher-Smith JA, Walter FM, Emery JD, et al. Risk prediction models for colorectal cancer: a systematic review. Cancer Prev Res (Phila) 2016;9(1):13–26.
38. Freedman AN, Slattery ML, Ballard-Barbash R, et al. Colorectal cancer risk prediction tool for white men and women without known susceptibility. J Clin Oncol 2009;27(5):686–93.
39. Park Y, Freedman AN, Gail MH, et al. Validation of a colorectal cancer risk prediction model among white patients age 50 years and older. J Clin Oncol 2009;27(5): 694–8.
40. Optenberg SA, Clark JY, Brawer MK, et al. Development of a decision-making tool to predict risk of prostate cancer: the cancer of the prostate risk index (capri) test. Urology 1997;50(5):665–72.
41. Thompson I, Thompson IM, Ankerst DP, et al. Assessing prostate cancer risk: results from the prostate cancer prevention trial. J Natl Cancer Inst 2006;98(8): 529–34.
42. Bruner DW, Baffoe-Bonnie A, Miller S, et al. Prostate cancer risk assessment program. A model for the early detection of prostate cancer. Oncology (Williston Park) 1999;13(3):325–34.
43. Kranse R, Roobol M, Schröder FH. A graphical device to represent the outcomes of a logistic regression analysis. Prostate 2008;68(15):1674–80.
44. Cruz M, Covinsky K, Widera EW, et al. Predicting 10-year mortality for older adults. JAMA 2013;309(9):874–6.
45. Schonberg MA, Davis RB, McCarthy EP, et al. External validation of an index to predict up to 9-year mortality of community-dwelling adults aged 65 and older. J Am Geriatr Soc 2011;59(8):1444–51.
46. Studenski S, Perera S, Patel K, et al. Gait speed and survival in older adults. JAMA 2011;305(1):50–8.
47. Charlson ME, Pompei P, Ales KL, et al. A new method of classifying prognostic comorbidity in longitudinal studies: development and validation. J Chronic Dis 1987;40(5):373–83.

48. Hall WH, Ramachandran R, Narayan S, et al. An electronic application for rapidly calculating Charlson Comorbidity Score. BMC Cancer 2004;4(4):94.
49. Lee SJ, Boscardin WJ, Stijacic-Cenzer I, et al. Time lag to benefit after screening for breast and colorectal cancer: meta-analysis of survival data from the United States, Sweden, United Kingdom, and Denmark. BMJ 2013;346:e8441.
50. Harris RP, Wilt TJ, Qaseem A, et al. A value framework for cancer screening: advice for high-value care from the American College of Physicians. Ann Intern Med 2015;162(10):712–7.
51. Herrera AP, Snipes SA, King DW, et al. Disparate inclusion of older adults in clinical trials: priorities and opportunities for policy and practice change. Am J Public Health 2010;100(S1):S105–12.
52. Saini SD, Vijan S, Schoenfeld P, et al. Role of quality measurement in inappropriate use of screening for colorectal cancer: retrospective cohort study. BMJ 2014;348:g1247.
53. Schwartz LM, Woloshin S, Fowler FJ, et al. Enthusiasm for cancer screening in the United States. JAMA 2004;291(1):71–8.
54. Zipkin DA, Umscheid CA, Keating NL, et al. Evidence-based risk communication. Ann Intern Med 2014;161(4):270.
55. Schoenborn NL, Bowman TL, Cayea D, et al. Primary care practitioners' views on incorporating long-term prognosis in the care of older adults. JAMA Intern Med 2016;176(5):671–8.
56. Pollack CE, Platz EA, Bhavsar NA, et al. Primary care providers' perspectives on discontinuing prostate cancer screening. Cancer 2012;118(22):5518–24.

Frailty Screening and Interventions

Considerations for Clinical Practice

Jeremy Walston, MD*, Brian Buta, MHS, Qian-Li Xue, PhD

KEYWORDS

• Frailty • Clinical • Assessment • Screening • Prevention • Intervention

KEY POINTS

- Frailty is a recognized health problem among older adults and vulnerable populations that increases the risk of adverse outcomes, including falls, hospitalization, and death.
- Multiple instruments exist to screen for frailty in clinical settings and more research is needed to validate these instruments beyond their predictive value.
- Frailty interventions include exercises, nutrition, and multicomponent strategies, though findings to date have been mixed.
- Preventing frailty is an important area for further research.

INTRODUCTION TO FRAILTY

Over the past 100 years, advances in medicine and public health have led to a nearly 2-fold increase in average lifespan.[1] Approximately 8.5% of the global population is 65 years or older, and this will increase to an estimated 16.7% by 2050.[2] Many health problems are related to aging, including chronic diseases, infections, disability, falls, and cognitive disorders.[2] There also seems to be a trend for increased vulnerability to health risks and poor outcomes as humans age.

Frailty has been viewed as a cornerstone of geriatric medicine and a platform of biological vulnerability to a host of other geriatric syndromes and adverse health outcomes.[3] Using a common frailty assessment instrument, an estimated 15% of noninstitutionalized adults in the United States are frail,[4] and global estimates of frailty range from 3.5% to 27.3%.[5] Clinical perspectives on the definition of frailty were initially broad; in the 1980s, chronologic age, care requirements, and disability were used

Disclosure Statement: The authors have nothing to disclose.
Johns Hopkins University Older Americans Independence Center, Johns Hopkins Asthma and Allergy Center, 5501 Hopkins Bayview Circle, Room 1A.62, Baltimore, MD 21224, USA
* Corresponding author. JHAAC Rm. 1A.62, 5501 Bayview Circle, Baltimore, MD 21217.
E-mail address: jwalston@jhmi.edu

Clin Geriatr Med 34 (2018) 25–38
https://doi.org/10.1016/j.cger.2017.09.004
0749-0690/18/© 2017 Elsevier Inc. All rights reserved.

geriatric.theclinics.com

synonymously with frailty.[6] In the following decade, clinical definitions became more refined though still included a wide range of domains.[7] The topic of frailty began receiving serious attention in the medical literature in the 1990s, as a reflection of the unexplained vulnerable state of older patients commonly observed by health care providers. Several key theoretic papers on frailty emerged during this time,[8–10] as did early operational definitions.[7] In 1992, Buchner and Wagner[8] discussed 3 components central to frailty: neurologic control, mechanical performance, and energy metabolism. In the same year, Fried,[9] in summarizing a workshop on the physiologic basis of frailty, described the syndromic nature of frailty with specific components, including weakness, fear of falling, and weight loss. This conference also distinguished frailty and disability as separate entities.

Fried and Walston[3] proposed the frailty phenotype with 5 components interlinked to form a cycle of frailty: weakness, slowness, exhaustion, low activity, and weight loss. Fried and colleagues[11] defined frailty "as a biologic syndrome of decreased reserve and resistance to stressors, resulting from cumulative declines across multiple physiologic systems, and causing vulnerability to adverse outcomes," and operationalized it using the frailty phenotype. The deficit accumulation approach emerged during the same period, which included counts of diseases, conditions, and comorbidities across many domains to determine frailty status.[12] More recently, a geriatric clinic in France has implemented a frailty screening tool based on the frailty phenotype that includes social and cognitive factors, along with physical components.[13] In 2013, members of a consensus group reached agreement on the following definition of frailty, "A medical syndrome with multiple causes and contributors that is characterized by diminished strength, endurance, and reduced physiologic function that increases an individual's vulnerability for developing increased dependency and/or death."[14]

Frailty Screening Instruments

Over the past 20 years, dozens, if not hundreds, of frailty assessment instruments have been developed and in part validated by showing the association between frailty and adverse health outcomes in older adults.[15] Most of these instruments are either (1) frailty phenotype instruments, in which motor and activity measures predominate and lead to an aggregate score that spans from robust to frail; or (2) frailty index instruments, in which comorbidities, social factors, psychological conditions, and function and cognitive decline measures are incorporated into an index in which the higher the number of conditions, the higher the frailty score.[16] Many frailty instruments are useful for identifying individuals at high risk for adverse outcomes but less so at informing clinical practice or the development of clinical interventions to prevent or treat frailty. Additionally, agreement between these instruments has been shown to vary greatly.[17] Maintaining validity in terms of ensuring that instruments are measuring their intended frailty-related constructs is another important consideration.[18–20]

Because short and simple instruments are most feasible in clinical practice, several quick screening tools have been developed and validated.[14] These include the Clinical Frailty Scale (CFS)[21] and the Fatigue, Resistance, Ambulation, Illnesses, and Loss of Weight (FRAIL) scale.[22] The CFS is based on clinical observation by the physician and assigns a score between 1 and 7 based on activity, function, and disability. The FRAIL scale is based on self-reported fatigue, mobility, strength, and weight loss, as well as a tally of the number of comorbidities. These 2 scales are especially relevant in clinical practice and require only a few minutes. The frailty phenotype and the Gérontopôle screening tool have also been recommended for screening purposes,[14] along with gait speed, as a single screening measure.[23]

Published best practice guidelines for recognizing and managing frailty in older adults in the United Kingdom highlighted 3 measures for rapid identification of frailty: gait speed less than 0.8 m/s, timed up-and-go test greater than 10s, and a score of greater than or equal to 3 on the Program of Research to Integrate Services for the Maintenance of Autonomy questionnaire.[24] Common clinical presentations, such as falls, delirium, and sudden immobility, may also indicate the presence of frailty in older adults.[24] Though quick identification tools are important in the clinical setting, caution must be advised because instruments are not necessarily interchangeable given the different items measured.[19] Also, there is frequent lack of agreement in identifying persons who are frail versus nonfrail persons when using these different assessment instruments.[24] **Table 1** provides a summary of selected tools that can be used for frailty screening.

SCREENING FOR FRAILTY IN THE CLINICAL SETTING

Frailty is associated with greater prevalence of adverse health outcomes, including mortality, disability, worsening mobility, falls, and hospitalization in the US population[4]; and it is predictive of these outcomes in epidemiologic cohorts.[11,20] Frailty, therefore, may be useful for risk prediction and decision-making in clinical settings. In a literature review that cataloged frailty instruments and their uses, however, the use of frailty assessment for clinical decision-making with regard to care delivery and management was found to be rare.[15] This low level of utilization in clinical decision making may reflect (1) lack of evidence and guidance on how to incorporate frailty status information within specific clinical settings and (2) confusion over which frailty instrument to select in a given specialty. In the following sections, studies of the use of frailty assessment in clinical settings are reviewed, the potential of frailty to provide value-added utility to clinical specialties is explored, and ongoing challenges and opportunities identified.

Screening for Frailty in General Clinical Practice

Despite disagreement on the best methodology to identify frailty in older adults, there has been an emerging trend toward the recognition of potential importance of screening for frailty to assist in general decision-making.[14,22,24] For example, screening for frailty has been recommended as an easy way to identify those older adults who would most benefit from a comprehensive geriatric assessment (CGA).[24] Recently, other guidelines have been proposed for older adults with diabetes in which glycemic targets of treatment differ depending on frailty status, with less stringent glycemic control recommended for frail older adults, whose compromised physiologic reserves may increase the risk of treatment-related adverse outcomes, such as hypoglycemia events.[25] Another example from the primary care setting includes ongoing research to ascertain whether or not frailty status should influence blood pressure target levels given that potential benefits may be offset by potential side effects of pharmacotherapy.[26,27]

Screening for Frailty in Subspecialty Populations

To date, frailty assessment has been used in a variety of clinical specialties for the identification of those at highest risk for adverse outcomes and for risk stratification to assist in clinical decision making.[28] **Table 2** is a summary from among a selected group of medical specialties: cardiology, infectious diseases, nephrology, oncology, and surgery.

Table 1
Selected instruments for frailty screening

Instrument	Components	Scoring
CFS[14,21]	Clinical judgment, ranging from very fit to severely frail: 1 = very fit; 2 = well; 3 = well, with treated comorbid disease; 4 = apparently vulnerable; 5 = mildly frail (some dependence on others for instrumental activities of daily living); 6 = moderately frail (help needed with instrumental and noninstrumental activities of daily living); 7 = severely frail (total dependence on others for activities of daily living or terminally ill)	Physician assigns score of 1–7 based on clinical judgment Physicians making the initial assessment given access to diagnoses and assessments related to these variables and other measures of comorbidity, function, and associated features that inform clinical judgments about the severity of frailty A secondary review and scoring is performed by a multidisciplinary team
FRAIL Scale[14,22]	Self-reported fatigue, resistance (ability to climb a single flight of stairs), ambulation (ability to walk 1 block), illnesses (more than 5), loss of weight (more than 5%)	Score range 0–5 No frailty = 0 deficits Intermediate frailty = 1 or 2 deficits Frailty = 3 or more deficits
Frailty Phenotype[11,14]	5 criteria: weight loss, measured weakness, self-reported exhaustion, measured slowness, low activity; questionnaire	Score range 0–5 Frail: ≥3 criteria present Intermediate or prefrail: 1 or 2 criteria present Robust or nonfrail: 0 criteria present
Gait Speed (as a single measure)[23,24]	Measured gait speed over 4 m	Gait speed <0.8 m/s is cutpoint for increased risk of adverse health outcomes Gait speed <0.2 m/s is cutpoint for extreme frailty

Gérontopôle Frailty Screening Tool[13,14]	6 questions to be answered by the practitioner or clinician: (1) whether the patient lives alone, (2) whether the patient has lost weight, (3) whether the patient has felt more tired, (4) whether the patient has memory problems, (5) whether the patient has found it difficult to get around, and (6) whether the patient has a slow gait (<1 m/s)	If the practitioner or clinician answer yes to any 1 of the 6 questions, the screening questionnaire asks for their clinical judgment on whether the patient is frail: if yes, a follow-up question is to be completed about to whether the patient is willing to be fully evaluated for frailty
PRISMA Questionnaire[24,56]	7 yes-or-no self-reported questions about: (1) age, (2) sex, (3) health problems that require a limit on activities, (4) help needed from someone regularly, (5) health problems that require one to stay at home, (6) having someone to court on if needed, and (7) regular use of an assistive device for walking	Answering yes to 3 of more of the 7 questions = potential disabilities or frailty
Timed Up-and-Go Test[24,57]	Measures of functional mobility (chair stair, 10-foot walk, and return the chair)	Frail = taking >10 s to complete the test

Abbreviation: PRISMA, Preferred Reporting Items for Systematic Reviews and Meta-Analyses.

Table 2
Frailty assessment in clinical research studies among medical specialties

Specialty	Frailty Prevalence	Instruments Used	Findings
Cardiology	10% to 60% among older adults with cardiovascular disease (CVD)[58]	Gait speed as a single measure, the frailty phenotype, and the CFS[58]	• 2-fold increase in mortality for frail older CVD patients across a broad spectrum of cardiovascular pathologic conditions and therapies[58] • Used as a component of patient selection for invasive and potentially high-risk therapies[59]
Infectious disease: human immunodeficiency virus (HIV)	15% among HIV-infected drug users; 10% among persons with AIDS-defining illness, after initiating combination antiretroviral therapy (cART)[60]	Modified version of the frailty phenotypes, the frailty index, and the Veterans Aging Cohort Study index[61]	• 3-fold increase in mortality for frail HIV-infected adults, independent of comorbidity and HIV disease stage[60] • Worse prognosis (AIDS, death) for HIV-infected adults with frailty before initiating cART than for those without pre-cART frailty[62]
Nephrology	Average of 36.8% among middle-aged to older adults with end-stage renal disease (ESRD)[63]	Modified version of the frailty phenotype[63]	• Among patients with ESRD, frailty is associated with falls,[64] mortality, hospitalization,[65] and health-related quality of life[66] • Frailty information may help to guide which ESRD patients are determined to be most suitable for kidney transplant[67]

Oncology	42% median (range 6%–86%) among older cancer patients[68]	Physical functional performance and the Vulnerable Elders Survey used to screen for patients who would most benefit from a full CGA[68,69]	• Frailty is predictive of all-cause and postoperative mortality, chemotherapy intolerance, and postoperative complications in cancer patients[68] • Routine frailty (and fitness) assessments can help guide treatment[68] and frailty is associated with cancer treatment recommendations[70]
Surgery	41.8%–50.3% among older patients undergoing elective cardiac and noncardiac surgery[71]	Frailty phenotype, Deficit Accumulation Index, and Edmonton Frail Scale[71,72]	• Utility of frailty has been proposed for several purposes: preoperative risk assessment, trauma triage, prehabilitation to modify risk, tailored anesthesia administration, team-based care options, delirium prevention, and decision-making for palliative care[73] • In preoperative risk assessment, recent studies have shown that frailty predicts postoperative outcomes in older patients receiving elective surgery or kidney transplant (regarded as internal stressors), even after accounting for the conventional measures used in preoperative risk assessment[72,74,75]

Challenges and Emerging Areas in Screening for Frailty

Despite calls to intensify efforts to screen for frailty among older adults,[14,29] a recognized need exists for further research on the contribution of frailty assessment to patient care and on best practices for managing frail patients. A study by Sourial and colleagues[30] found a significant but modest added predictive value of frailty markers for disability, beyond the common clinical markers of age, sex, and chronic diseases. Therefore, before clinical frailty screening can be implemented without reservation, more studies examining the net contribution of frailty screening to risk prediction in different settings and populations, and for both clinical and patient-centered outcomes, are needed.

A notable emerging area for frailty screening is the use of biomarkers to identify frail older adults.[31–33] However, several issues remain; a consensus effort to reach agreement on a definition of frailty for clinical uses found a significant disagreement on the selection of specific biomarkers for frailty, especially laboratory-based markers.[34] One area of agreement is that no single biomarker may be adequate for frailty prediction or diagnosis.[34] Currently, efforts are underway to develop methods for identifying multivariate approaches to biomarker models for frailty.[35]

INTERVENTIONS FOR FRAILTY AND PREVENTING THE DEVELOPMENT OF FRAILTY
Frailty Interventions

Interventions for frailty have been proposed along a spectrum of frail health (**Fig. 1**). Four major types of intervention to improve health outcomes of frail individuals or, most recently, combat frailty itself have been attempted: exercises, nutritional intervention, multicomponent interventions, and individually tailored geriatric care models. Most of the exercise interventions focused on flexibility, balance, resistance, and endurance training. The results varied by the type, duration, and modality of interventions, gender, residential status, study outcomes, and frailty assessment tools used.[36] The oldest old, frail women, or those living in long-term care facilities tend to benefit the most.[36] A progressive exercise program beginning with flexibility and balancing training, followed by resistance and endurance training has shown to be effective in improving physical function; and the gradual increase of exercise intensity may be particularly appealing to sedentary frail older adults with safety concerns and difficulty with compliance. In fact, the most recent updated American College of Sports Medicine guidelines[37] recommend that resistance and/or balance training should precede aerobic training for this population.

Very few studies have directly evaluated the impact of exercise intervention on frailty itself, other than its components or physical function in general.[38] The Lifestyle Interventions and Independence for Elders pilot (LIFE-P) study reported that a 12-month physical activity intervention was associated with 9% lower frailty prevalence, and significantly greater reduction in the mean number of frailty criteria for blacks and those with frailty at baseline relative to a successful aging education group. However, the trends observed in the LIFE-P were primarily driven by intervention-related change in sedentary behavior suggest that interventions designed to target the phenotypic components of frailty, such as muscle weakness and inactivity, may not be sufficient for addressing or alleviating the root causes of frailty.

In the domain of nutrition, a recent review by Manal and colleagues[39] summarized findings of 4 types of intervention: specific nutritional supplement formula; daily food fortification with protein supplement; nutritional education and counseling; and supplementation of micronutrients, including vitamin D, omega-3 fatty acids, and multivitamins. The results have been mixed due to the type and duration of nutrition

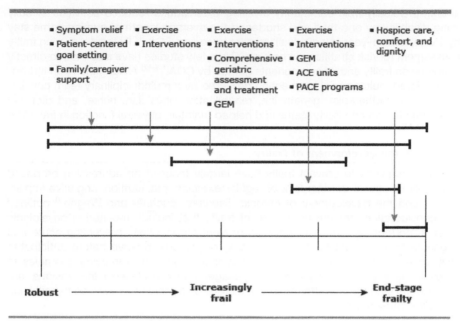

- Symptom relief
- Patient-centered goal setting
- Family/caregiver support

- Exercise
- Interventions

- Exercise
- Interventions
- Comprehensive geriatric assessment and treatment
- GEM

- Exercise
- Interventions
- GEM
- ACE units
- PACE programs

- Hospice care, comfort, and dignity

Robust   →   Increasingly frail   →   End-stage frailty

Fig. 1. Potential interventions along the spectrum of frailty in older adults. (*Reproduced with permission from* Walston JD. Frailty. In: UpToDate, Post TW (Ed), UpToDate, Waltham, MA. (Accessed August 22, 2017.) Copyright © 2017 UpToDate, Inc. For more information visit www.uptodate.com. and *Modified from* Walston JD, Fried LP. Frailty and its implications for care. In: Morrison RS, Meire DE, editors. Geriatric palliative care. New York: Oxford University Press; 2003. p. 101; with permission.)

intervention and nutritional status before the intervention. For example, food fortification,[40] multinutrient supplementation,[41] and vitamin D[42] showed no significant effect, whereas other studies of nutritional supplementation reported reversal of weight loss and improved nutritional status but not functional outcomes such as grip strength. The latter findings led to the hypothesis that nutritional intervention alone may be too little, and too late, to reverse the process of decreased muscle strength and functional decline.[43] Nutritional advice and counseling[44,45] improved frailty status only among older adults at risk for malnutrition.[46]

Because of the likely multifactorial etiologic factors underlying frailty, interventions combining exercise, behavioral therapy, nutrition, and cognitive training have also been tested. For example, the combination of exercise and nutrition intervention resulted in frailty status improvement[47–49] or reduction in prefrailty-to-frailty transition.[50] Most recently, a 6-month trial combining nutritional supplementation, physical training, and cognitive training was found to improve frailty status in groups receiving each treatment alone, as well as in the group receiving all 3, and the improvement persisted 6 months after treatment cessation.[51]

Besides efforts to identify a specific intervention or combinations of intervention that are uniformly efficacious for all frail older adults, individually tailored interventions based on impairments identified by the CGA have received growing attention. Although evidence on the effectiveness of CGA in preventing functional decline is mixed in the general population, some have argued that the value of CGA could be greater in frail older adults at high risk for functional decline. Consistent with this hypothesis, a 6-month prehabilitation program for the prevention of functional decline among physically frail, community-dwelling older adults reduced activities of daily living disability by one-third and shortened the average length of nursing home stay by 1 week after 1-year of individualized care based on CGA.[52] Rather than using frailty assessment for risk stratification before CGA, a few studies have also tried to directly intervene on frailty and its components guided by CGA.[53–55] Among them, an individually tailored multifactorial intervention delivered by a multidisciplinary team consisting of a physiotherapist, geriatrician, rehabilitation physician, nurse, and dietician was found to improve frailty status and helped maintain physical function in frail older adults.[54,55]

Preventing the Development of Frailty

Recommendations to prevent frailty have largely focused on addressing proposed drivers of functional decline: lack of regular exercise, malnutrition, cognitive impairments, and the development of chronic diseases. Buchner and Wagner[8] outlined key considerations for the prevention of frailty that include monitoring physiologic reserve, performing regular exercise to prevent chronic loss, preventing acute and subacute loss (ie, vaccinations), increasing physiologic reserve before anticipated loss (prehabilitation before an elective hospitalization), and removing obstacles to recovery (using geriatric evaluation and management). As detailed in the previous section, several studies have attempted to intervene on factors that may lead to frailty and its clinical presentation.

SUMMARY

Screening for frailty in clinical settings sits at an interesting crossroads. In some arenas, frailty assessments are already being carried out routinely in geriatric clinics and in certain medical specialties. Notably, in these specialty populations, frailty has shown promising utility in identifying patients who may have poor outcomes following treatment or who may require prehabilitation before a procedure. On the other hand, cautions have been raised against rushing to implement frailty in general clinical settings due to (1) the lack of an agreed-on operational definition of frailty, which, in turn, may results in misclassification; (2) the need for further research on its added clinical value; and (3) the need for evidence-based guidelines on how to manage, treat, and in some cases reverse frailty in patients. As the world's population of older adults increases rapidly, the benefits and ongoing challenges related to frailty assessment will become a priority for more and more health care providers.

REFERENCES

1. National Institute on Aging and World Health Organization. Global Health and Aging. 2011. Available at: https://www.nia.nih.gov/research/publication/global-health-and-aging/living-longer. Accessed June 15, 2017.
2. He W, Goodkind D, Kowal P. An aging world: 2015. International population reports, P95/16–1. In: Bureau USC, editor. Washington, DC: U.S. Government Publishing Office; 2016. Available at: https://www.census.gov/content/dam/Census/library/publications/2016/demo/p95-16-1.pdf. Accessed July 5, 2017.
3. Fried LP, Walston J. Frailty and failure to thrive. In: Hazzard WR, et al, editors. Principles of geriatric medicine and gerontology, vol. 4. New York: McGraw Hill; 1998. p. 1387–402.
4. Bandeen-Roche K, Seplaki CL, Huang J, et al. Frailty in older adults: a nationally representative profile in the United States. J Gerontol A Biol Sci Med Sci 2015;70: 1427–34.

5. Xue QL, Buta B, Varadhan R, et al. Frailty and geriatric syndromes. In: Satariano WA, Maus M, editors. Aging, place, and health: a global perspective. Burlington (MA): Jones & Bartlett Learning; 2017. p. 191–230.
6. Hogan DB, MacKnight C, Bergman H, Steering Committee, Canadian Initiative on Frailty and Aging. Models, definitions, and criteria of frailty. Aging Clin Exp Res 2003;15:1–29.
7. Winograd CH, Gerety MB, Chung M, et al. Screening for frailty: criteria and predictors of outcomes. J Am Geriatr Soc 1991;39:778–84.
8. Buchner DM, Wagner EH. Preventing frail health. Clin Geriatr Med 1992;8:1–17.
9. Fried LP. Conference on the physiologic basis of frailty. April 28, 1992, Baltimore, Maryland, U.S.A. Introduction. Aging (Milano) 1992;4:251–2.
10. Bortz WM 2nd. The physics of frailty. J Am Geriatr Soc 1993;41:1004–8.
11. Fried LP, Tangen CM, Walston J, et al. Frailty in older adults: evidence for a phenotype. J Gerontol A Biol Sci Med Sci 2001;56:M146–56.
12. Mitnitski AB, Mogilner AJ, Rockwood K. Accumulation of deficits as a proxy measure of aging. ScientificWorldJournal 2001;1:323–36.
13. Subra J, Gillette-Guyonnet S, Cesari M, et al. The integration of frailty into clinical practice: preliminary results from the Gerontopole. J Nutr Health Aging 2012;16: 714–20.
14. Morley JE, Vellas B, van Kan GA, et al. Frailty consensus: a call to action. J Am Med Dir Assoc 2013;14:392–7.
15. Buta BJ, Walston JD, Godino JG, et al. Frailty assessment instruments: systematic characterization of the uses and contexts of highly-cited instruments. Ageing Res Rev 2016;26:53–61.
16. Walston JD, Bandeen-Roche K. Frailty: a tale of two concepts. BMC Med 2015; 13:185.
17. Aguayo GA, Donneau AF, Vaillant MT, et al. Agreement between 35 published frailty scores in the general population. Am J Epidemiol 2017;186(4):1–15.
18. Rockwood K. What would make a definition of frailty successful? Age Ageing 2005;34:432–4.
19. Xue QL, Varadhan R. What is missing in the validation of frailty instruments? J Am Med Dir Assoc 2014;15:141–2.
20. Bandeen-Roche K, Xue QL, Ferrucci L, et al. Phenotype of frailty: characterization in the women's health and aging studies. J Gerontol A Biol Sci Med Sci 2006;61: 262–6.
21. Rockwood K, Song X, MacKnight C, et al. A global clinical measure of fitness and frailty in elderly people. CMAJ 2005;173:489–95.
22. Abellan van Kan G, Rolland Y, Bergman H, et al. The I.A.N.A Task Force on frailty assessment of older people in clinical practice. J Nutr Health Aging 2008;12: 29–37.
23. Abellan Van Kan G, Rolland Y, Andrieu S, et al. Gait speed at usual pace as a predictor of adverse outcomes in community-dwelling older people: an International Academy on Nutrition and Aging (IANA) Task Force. J Nutr Health Aging 2009;13:881–9.
24. Turner G, Clegg A, British Geriatrics Society, Age UK, Royal College of General Practioners. Best practice guidelines for the management of frailty: a British Geriatrics Society, Age UK and Royal College of General Practitioners report. Age Ageing 2014;43:744–7.
25. Meneilly GS, Knip A, Tessier D, Canadian Diabetes Association Clinical Practice Guidelines Expert Committee. Diabetes in the elderly. Can J Diabetes 2013; 37(Suppl 1):S184–90.

26. Williamson JDSM, Applegate WB, Berlowitz DR, et al, SPRINT Research Group. Intensive vs standard blood pressure control and cardiovascular disease outcomes in adults aged ≥75 years: a randomized clinical trial. JAMA 2016;315: 2673–82.
27. Pajewski NM, Williamson JD, Applegate WB, et al. Characterizing frailty status in the systolic blood pressure intervention trial. J Gerontol A Biol Sci Med Sci 2016; 71:649–55.
28. Walston J, Robinson TN, Zieman S, et al. Integrating frailty research into the medical specialties-report from a U13 conference. J Am Geriatr Soc 2017;2134–9.
29. Vellas B, Cestac P, Moley JE. Implementing frailty into clinical practice: we cannot wait. J Nutr Health Aging 2012;16:599–600.
30. Sourial N, Bergman H, Karunananthan S, et al. Implementing frailty into clinical practice: a cautionary tale. J Gerontol A Biol Sci Med Sci 2013;68:1505–11.
31. Garcia-Garcia FJ, Carcaillon L, Fernandez-Tresguerres J, et al. A new operational definition of frailty: the Frailty Trait Scale. J Am Med Dir Assoc 2014;15:371.e7-13.
32. King KE, Fillenbaum GG, Cohen HJ. A cumulative deficit laboratory test-based frailty index: personal and neighborhood associations. J Am Geriatr Soc 2017; 65(9):1981–7.
33. Walston JD. Connecting age-related biological decline to frailty and late-life vulnerability. Nestle Nutr Inst Workshop Ser 2015;83:1–10.
34. Rodriguez-Manas L, Feart C, Mann G, et al. Searching for an operational definition of frailty: a Delphi method based consensus statement. The frailty operative definition-consensus conference project. J Gerontol A Biol Sci Med Sci 2013;68: 62–7.
35. Calvani R, Marini F, Cesari M, et al. Biomarkers for physical frailty and sarcopenia: state of the science and future developments. J Cachexia Sarcopenia Muscle 2015;6:278–86.
36. Theou O, Stathokostas L, Roland KP, et al. The effectiveness of exercise interventions for the management of frailty: a systematic review. J Aging Res 2011;2011: 569194.
37. Chodzko-Zajko WJ, Proctor DN, Fiatarone Singh MA, et al. American College of Sports Medicine position stand. Exercise and physical activity for older adults. Med Sci Sports Exerc 2009;41:1510–30.
38. Puts MT, Toubasi S, Andrew MK, et al. Interventions to prevent or reduce the level of frailty in community-dwelling older adults: a scoping review of the literature and international policies. Age Ageing 2017;383–92.
39. Manal B, Suzana S, Singh DK. Nutrition and frailty: a review of clinical intervention studies. J Frailty Aging 2015;4:100–6.
40. Smoliner C, Norman K, Scheufele R, et al. Effects of food fortification on nutritional and functional status in frail elderly nursing home residents at risk of malnutrition. Nutrition 2008;24:1139–44.
41. Fiatarone MA, O'Neill EF, Ryan ND, et al. Exercise training and nutritional supplementation for physical frailty in very elderly people. N Engl J Med 1994;330: 1769–75.
42. Latham NK, Anderson CS, Lee A, et al. A randomized, controlled trial of quadriceps resistance exercise and vitamin D in frail older people: the Frailty Interventions Trial in Elderly Subjects (FITNESS). J Am Geriatr Soc 2003;51:291–9.
43. Payette H, Boutier V, Coulombe C, et al. Benefits of nutritional supplementation in free-living, frail, undernourished elderly people: a prospective randomized community trial. J Am Diet Assoc 2002;102:1088–95.

44. Rydwik E, Frandin K, Akner G, et al. Effects of a physical training and nutritional intervention program in frail elderly people regarding habitual physical activity level and activities of daily living–a randomized controlled pilot study. Arch Gerontol Geriatr 2010;51:283–9.
45. Lammes E, Rydwik E, Akner G, et al. Effects of nutritional intervention and physical training on energy intake, resting metabolic rate and body composition in frail elderly. A randomised, controlled pilot study. J Nutr Health Aging 2012;16:162–7.
46. Nykänen I, Rissanen TH, Sulkava R, et al. Effects of individual dietary counseling as part of a comprehensive geriatric assessment (CGA) on nutritional status: a population-based intervention study. J Nutr Health Aging 2014;18:54–8.
47. Chan DCD, Tsou HH, Yang RS, et al. A pilot randomized controlled trial to improve geriatric frailty. BMC Geriatr 2012;12:58.
48. Kim H, Suzuki T, Kim M, et al. Effects of exercise and milk fat globule membrane (MFGM) supplementation on body composition, physical function, and hematological parameters in community-dwelling frail Japanese women: a randomized double blind, placebo-controlled, follow-up trial. PLoS One 2015;10:e0116256.
49. Tarazona-Santabalbina FJ, Gomez-Cabrera MC, Perez-Ros P, et al. A multicomponent exercise intervention that reverses frailty and improves cognition, emotion, and social networking in the community-dwelling frail elderly: a randomized clinical trial. J Am Med Dir Assoc 2016;17:426–33.
50. Serra-Prat M, Sist X, Domenich R, et al. Effectiveness of an intervention to prevent frailty in pre-frail community-dwelling older people consulting in primary care: a randomised controlled trial. Age Ageing 2017;401–7.
51. Ng TP, Feng L, Nyunt MSZ, et al. Nutritional, physical, cognitive, and combination interventions and frailty reversal among older adults: a randomized controlled trial. Am J Med 2015;128:1225.
52. Gill TM, Baker DI, Gottschalk M, et al. A prehabilitation program for the prevention of functional decline: evidence for an expanded benefit. J Am Geriatr Soc 2003;51:S36–7.
53. Li CM, Chen CY, Li CY, et al. The effectiveness of a comprehensive geriatric assessment intervention program for frailty in community-dwelling older people: a randomized, controlled trial. Arch Gerontol Geriatr 2010;50(Suppl 1):S39–42.
54. Cameron ID, Fairhall N, Langron C, et al. A multifactorial interdisciplinary intervention reduces frailty in older people: randomized trial. BMC Med 2013;11:65.
55. Fairhall N, Sherrington C, Cameron ID, et al. A multifactorial intervention for frail older people is more than twice as effective among those who are compliant: complier average causal effect analysis of a randomised trial. J Physiother 2017;63:40–4.
56. Raiche M, Hebert R, Dubois MF. PRISMA-7: a case-finding tool to identify older adults with moderate to severe disabilities. Arch Gerontol Geriatr 2008;47:9–18.
57. Podsiadlo D, Richardson S. The timed "Up & Go": a test of basic functional mobility for frail elderly persons. J Am Geriatr Soc 1991;39:142–8.
58. Afilalo J, Alexander KP, Mack MJ, et al. Frailty assessment in the cardiovascular care of older adults. J Am Coll Cardiol 2014;63:747–62.
59. Sepehri A, Beggs T, Hassan A, et al. The impact of frailty on outcomes after cardiac surgery: a systematic review. J Thorac Cardiovasc Surg 2014;148:3110–7.
60. Piggott DA, Varadhan R, Mehta SH, et al. Frailty, inflammation, and mortality among persons aging with HIV infection and injection drug use. J Gerontol A Biol Sci Med Sci 2015;70:1542–7.

61. Piggott DA, Erlandson KM, Yarasheski KE. Frailty in HIV: epidemiology, biology, measurement, interventions, and research needs. Curr HIV/AIDS Rep 2016;13: 340–8.
62. Desquilbet L, Jacobson LP, Fried LP, et al. A frailty-related phenotype before HAART initiation as an independent risk factor for AIDS or death after HAART among HIV-infected men. J Gerontol A Biol Sci Med Sci 2011;66:1030–8.
63. Kojima G. Prevalence of frailty in end-stage renal disease: a systematic review and meta-analysis. Int Urol Nephrol 2017. [Epub ahead of print].
64. McAdams-DeMarco MA, Suresh S, Law A, et al. Frailty and falls among adult patients undergoing chronic hemodialysis: a prospective cohort study. BMC Nephrol 2013;14:224.
65. McAdams-DeMarco MA, Law A, Salter ML, et al. Frailty as a novel predictor of mortality and hospitalization in individuals of all ages undergoing hemodialysis. J Am Geriatr Soc 2013;61:896–901.
66. McAdams-DeMarco MA, Ying H, Olorundare I, et al. Frailty and health-related quality of life in end stage renal disease patients of all ages. J Frailty Aging 2016;5:174–9.
67. McAdams-DeMarco MA, Ying H, Olorundare I, et al. Individual frailty components and mortality in kidney transplant recipients. Transplantation 2017;101(9): 2126–213.
68. Handforth C, Clegg A, Young C, et al. The prevalence and outcomes of frailty in older cancer patients: a systematic review. Ann Oncol 2015;26:1091–101.
69. Hamaker ME, Jonker JM, de Rooij SE, et al. Frailty screening methods for predicting outcome of a comprehensive geriatric assessment in elderly patients with cancer: a systematic review. Lancet Oncol 2012;13:e437–44.
70. Farcet A, de Decker L, Pauly V, et al. Frailty markers and treatment decisions in patients seen in oncogeriatric clinics: results from the ASRO pilot study. PLoS One 2016;11:e0149732.
71. Partridge JS, Harari D, Dhesi JK. Frailty in the older surgical patient: a review. Age Ageing 2012;41:142–7.
72. Makary MA, Segev DL, Pronovost PJ, et al. Frailty as a predictor of surgical outcomes in older patients. J Am Coll Surg 2010;210:901–8.
73. Robinson TN, Walston JD, Brummel NE, et al. Frailty for surgeons: review of a national institute on aging conference on frailty for specialists. J Am Coll Surg 2015; 221:1083–92.
74. Garonzik-Wang JM, Govindan P, Grinnan JW, et al. Frailty and delayed graft function in kidney transplant recipients. Arch Surg 2012;147:190–3.
75. McAdams-DeMarco MA, Law A, Salter ML, et al. Frailty and early hospital readmission after kidney transplantation. Am J Transplant 2013;13:2091–5.

Screening for Medication Appropriateness in Older Adults

Andrew R. Zullo, PharmD, PhD[a], Shelly L. Gray, PharmD, MS[b],
Holly M. Holmes, MD, MS[c], Zachary A. Marcum, PharmD, PhD[b],*

KEYWORDS

- Elderly • Geriatrics • Deprescribing • Inappropriate prescribing • Polypharmacy

KEY POINTS

- Medication appropriateness is a critical issue in older adults, who are exposed to multiple medications and are more vulnerable to medication-related problems.
- Improving medication appropriateness needs to be addressed in all care settings; each care setting (community, hospital, nursing home) presents unique challenges and opportunities regarding appropriate medication use.
- Focused screening and intervention to improve medication appropriateness can be accomplished using readily available tools that can be integrated into clinical processes and, in some cases, into the electronic medical record.

INTRODUCTION

Medications are the most frequently used form of therapy for medical problems in older adults.[1] Older adults often have multiple medical conditions that may require several medications to manage.[2] Although pharmacotherapy can improve quality and quantity of life for older adults, there are also inherent risks. Of potential concern

Disclosure Statement: Drs A.R. Zullo and Z.A. Marcum are supported by awards from the Agency for Healthcare Research and Quality (5K12HS022998 and 5K12HS022982). Dr H.M. Holmes is supported by a grant from the Cancer Prevention and Research Institute of Texas (RP160674). Dr S.L. Gray is supported by awards from the National Institute on Aging (AG006781 and AG045050-03S1). The authors have no other relevant conflicts of interest to disclose.

[a] Department of Health Services, Policy, and Practice, Brown University School of Public Health, 121 South Main Street, Providence, RI 02912, USA; [b] Department of Pharmacy, University of Washington, School of Pharmacy, 1959 Northeast Pacific Street, Box 357630, Seattle, WA 98195, USA; [c] Division of Geriatric and Palliative Medicine, The University of Texas Health Science Center at Houston, McGovern Medical School, 6431 Fannin Street, MSB 5.116, Houston, TX 77030, USA
* Corresponding author.
E-mail address: zmarcum@uw.edu

Clin Geriatr Med 34 (2018) 39–54
https://doi.org/10.1016/j.cger.2017.09.003
geriatric.theclinics.com
0749-0690/18/© 2017 Elsevier Inc. All rights reserved.

is that inappropriate medication use can lead to medication-related problems, such as adverse drug reactions, therapeutic failures, and adverse drug withdrawal events.[3] These medication-related problems are associated with morbidity, mortality, and additional health care costs.

Medication appropriateness is a global concept composed of 3 specific domains: (1) overuse, (2) potentially inappropriate medication (PIM) use, and (3) underuse (**Table 1**). Overuse can be defined as the use of more medications than clinically needed. Examples of medication overuse include duplication of therapy (eg, use of 2 nonsteroidal anti-inflammatory drugs), use of medication with no medical indication (eg, proton pump inhibitor [PPI] without an indication), or use of a medication that is not effective. Overuse is frequently referred to as polypharmacy, although it is important to recognize that the target of screening is *unnecessary* polypharmacy.[4] The Screening Tool of Older Person's Prescriptions (STOPP) is explicit criteria organized by physiologic system along with explanations to help providers discontinue unnecessary medications (and those that are potentially inappropriate).[5,6] PIM use is defined as medication use where the risk outweighs the benefit. Most commonly, PIM use is assessed with explicit criteria, such as the American Geriatrics Society Beers Criteria for Potentially Inappropriate Medication Use in Older Adults, which are guidelines to help clinicians to maximize benefit and minimize harm when prescribing medications to older adults.[6,7] Underuse is the lack of medication therapy in those with a clinical indication based on guideline recommendations. It can be due to a host of reasons, including lack of sufficient evidence in older adults (because of their frequent exclusion from studies), inadequate insurance coverage, patient goals of care, and provider perception of the patient's prognosis, to name a few. Underuse can be assessed with explicit criteria like the Screening Tool to Alert doctors to Right Treatment (START) criteria, which is a validated tool that helps identify prescribing omissions by physiologic system.[6,8] **Table 2** provides clinical examples of types of prescribing problems by care setting.

Screening for appropriate medication use in older adults thus ideally involves the use of patient-level information and an up-to-date evidence base. For patient-level information, the following information is needed: (1) an accurate medical problem list, and (2) a comprehensive and up-to-date medication list, including prescription, over-the-counter, and supplement use. In addition, an up-to-date evidence base is needed in order to inform the identification and resolution of medication-related problems. Importantly, patient preferences should always be solicited and incorporated into such screening and any subsequent decision-making regarding pharmacotherapy.

Table 1 Three domains of medication appropriateness		
Domain	**Definition**	**Example Measures**
Overuse	Use of more medications than clinically necessary	Explicit: STOPP Implicit: MAI
PIM use	Use where the risk outweighs the benefit	Explicit: Beers Criteria/STOPP Implicit: MAI
Underuse	Absence of evidence-based medication use in those with a clinical indication	Explicit: START Implicit: AOU index

Abbreviations: AOU, assessment of underutilization; MAI, medication appropriateness index.

Care Setting	Medication Inappropriateness Type	Clinical Hypothetical Example
Community	Overuse	87 year-old woman living independently at home taking omeprazole and ranitidine for indigestion
	PIM use	76 year-old woman with a history of falls using acetaminophen/diphenhydramine for insomnia
	Underuse	65 year-old man with clinical atherosclerotic cardiovascular disease not receiving a high-intensity statin
Hospital	Overuse	76 year-old man with no indication for stress ulcer prophylaxis and no history of GERD receiving esomeprazole
	PIM use	66 year-old woman with opioid use disorder started on scheduled long-acting oxycodone on admission for osteoarthritis pain
	Underuse	68 year-old man with Parkinson disease whose levodopa was not continued while inpatient due to medication reconciliation error
Nursing home	Overuse	93 year-old woman with advanced cancer and poor prognosis receiving 16 scheduled medications, including a statin, bisphosphonate, calcium, and vitamin D
	PIM use	87 year-old woman with advanced dementia receiving risperidone for new-onset behavioral symptoms without aggression
	Underuse	74 year-old woman with osteoporosis and a history of major osteoporotic fracture not receiving a bisphosphonate

Table 2
Examples of medication inappropriateness across care settings in older adults

Abbreviation: GERD, gastroesophageal reflux disease.

The objectives of this review are as follows:

1. To describe the impact of medication inappropriateness on health outcomes and the rationale for performing screening;
2. To examine practical ways in which screening for medication appropriateness can be done across care settings;
3. To highlight gaps in knowledge and future research needs to inform clinical practice; and
4. To summarize clinical strategies to screen for medication appropriateness.

IMPACT OF MEDICATION INAPPROPRIATENESS ON HEALTH OUTCOMES

Inappropriate medication use in older adults has been shown to increase the risk of morbidity, mortality, and health care costs. Specifically, overuse, the use of more medications than are medically necessary,[9] has been shown to be associated with higher likelihood of unplanned hospitalization in older adults.[10,11] PIM use has been found to be associated with confusion, falls, and mortality.[7,12] Underuse has been found to be associated with unplanned hospitalization in older adults.[13] Furthermore, it has been estimated that for every dollar spent purchasing medications, approximately $1.75 is spent treating drug-related problems.[14,15] It is clear that medication-related problems are common and costly to older adults and the health care system.

RATIONALE FOR SCREENING FOR MEDICATION APPROPRIATENESS

The impact of overuse, PIM use, and underuse of medications on health outcomes is a strong part of the rationale for screening for medication appropriateness. Above and beyond that apparent clinical benefit, other potential benefits are likely to exist. We now function in an era of accountable care. In such an era, medication appropriateness screening is a potential high-impact opportunity to not only improve health but also reduce costs to the patient and health care system while improving patient satisfaction.

HOW TO SCREEN FOR MEDICATION APPROPRIATENESS
Overview

Screening for medication appropriateness may seem like a daunting task at first given that older adults often have multiple medical conditions and medications. This clinical complexity leads to many possible appropriate and inappropriate medication-condition and medication-medication combinations. Nonetheless, strategies for incorporating medication appropriateness screening into clinical practice can be efficient and feasible.

Targeted Reviews

One approach to screening is to select a specific therapeutic area or condition. This selection could be based on one or more criteria. Clinicians might select a condition for screening that is highly prevalent in the patient population they serve. For example, focusing on diabetes may narrow the scope of the medication appropriateness screening while addressing a condition of high relevance. Selecting a medication class to target for screening may also be a feasible first step. For instance, screening all patients on antipsychotics can allow for a targeted approach. Expertise of the clinicians in the primary care practice is another parameter for selecting a therapeutic area or condition for screening. If a practice has a pharmacist with prior training in infectious diseases, a focus on infectious illnesses might be a sensible way to initially implement screening. Furthermore, reimbursement is a prudent way to select a screening focus. Conditions included in Medicare's Hospital Readmissions Reduction Program are a common focus for screening.[16] Practices could therefore start by screening for medication appropriateness in patients with acute myocardial infarction, heart failure, and pneumonia. Finally, the preferences and care goals of patients may be an ideal starting place for the implementation of medication appropriateness screening. Patient visits could begin with a reappraisal of patients' goals of care and preferences. Medications could then be discontinued or initiated through shared decision making to maximally align the care plan with the patients' values. Two potential questions to ask patients are, "Do you think that you are currently taking too many medications?" and "Which of your medications do you feel is least beneficial to you?" Ultimately, deciding where to start will be determined based on resources, priorities, and quality measures.

Dashboards, Reports, and Electronic Medical Records

The use of dashboards and reports is another way to implement medication appropriateness screening. Dashboards have been successfully developed for patient management.[17–20] Dashboards are often condition-specific applications that attempt to provide timely and clinically relevant information for clinician decision making. For example, dashboards might display the number of PIMs that a patient is on or display those patients who are on any PIMs. Peterson and colleagues[21] conducted a pilot study of hospitalized adults aged 65 years and older in which they used a computerized PIMs dashboard to identify individuals with at least one administered PIM or a high calculated anticholinergic score. The dashboard was also able to show the 48-hour cumulative narcotic and benzodiazepine administration for each patient. Upon completion of the study, the investigators concluded that the dashboard provided an efficient mechanism for providers to perform medication appropriateness screening while older adults were hospitalized, and to subsequently deliver a point-of-care pharmacist intervention to improve medication use.[21] Dashboards are a promising method for medication appropriateness screening, but more evidence is needed to support their full integration.

Computerized decision support programs are being developed to implement inappropriate medication use criteria into clinical practice.[22,23] The inclusion of criteria into computerized decision support tools is relatively new. Although neither explicit criteria[5,7] nor computerized decision support[24] is new, combining these 2 approaches continues to increase in uptake over time.[25] For example, the STOPP tool was successfully integrated into a computer-based tool to reduce PIM use in an example published in 2016.[26] The investigators conducted an observational study of patients aged ≥65 years admitted to geriatric hospital units in Italy. They found that the computerized tool successfully enabled treating physicians to reduce PIM use. Other forthcoming studies have implemented the Beers Criteria medications as computerized decision support.[4] Until more information is available about the incorporation of explicit criteria into computerized decision support tools, standalone online tools and other resources may be a viable solution to assist with medication appropriateness screening.

Online Resources to Screen for Medication Appropriateness

Practices should incorporate tools into their daily workflow that provide structure for the process of medication appropriateness screening. Several resources exist to assist with screening for medication appropriateness and reduction of inappropriate medications (Table 3). All of the available resources aim to systematize the process of screening for medication appropriateness or to easily integrate processes to deprescribe inappropriate medications for primary care clinicians.

Most busy clinicians are likely to prefer interactive online tools because much of clinical practice now involves use of an electronic medical record (EMR) and online resources. MedStopper (http://medstopper.com/) is one such notable tool.[27] The tool focuses on deprescribing of medications and was designed with frail older patients in mind.[28] It is important to note that the MedStopper tool only addresses overuse and PIM use, not underuse. It is generally easy to use and intuitive. After indicating whether a patient is frail or not, the user then enters a drug and the condition for which it was prescribed. This process is repeated for each of the drugs that a patient is taking. The tool returns information on whether the drug is likely to improve symptoms, reduce the risk for future illness, and increase the risk for future harm. It also returns advice on tapering, which is especially popular among users.[28] No studies have confirmed that use of the tool can improve the efficiency of screening for medication appropriateness.

Utilization of Pharmacists

As medication experts, pharmacists (especially those trained in geriatrics) are ideally suited on the health care team to lead screening efforts for medication appropriateness in older adults.[29] Even without geriatrics training, pharmacists across all care settings can learn key principles of geriatric pharmacotherapy to apply to screening activities. One of the main components of screening for medication appropriateness

Table 3
Medication appropriateness resources

Problem	Tool	Type	Source	Link	Description	Pros	Cons
PIM use	Deprescribing Guidelines	Web site with downloadable materials	Canadian Deprescribing Network	http://deprescribing.org	Algorithms, patient information brochures, and pamphlets to promote deprescribing of proton pump inhibitors, benzodiazepines and sedative-hypnotics, and glucose-lowering agents	• Free • Written at appropriate health literacy levels for patient use • Evaluated in at least one clinical trial[43]	• Focused on only a few select classes of drugs
Overuse	A Practical Guide to Stopping Medicines in Older People	Article	*Best Practice Journal*	http://www.bpac.org.nz/BPJ/2010/April/stopguide.aspx	Article focused on (1) a framework of the factors to consider when deprescribing, including patient wishes, indication and benefit, appropriateness, duration of use, medication adherence, and the prescribing cascade and (2) stepwise guidance for deprescribing	• Contains specific guidance on safe tapering methods for specific drug classes	• Conceptual, less practical in busy clinical situations

Overuse and PIM use	Deprescribing Resources	Web resource with downloadable materials	Deprescribing Clinical Reference Group, the Australian Government, and Primary Health Tasmania	http://www.primaryhealthtas.com.au/resources/deprescribing	Downloadable fact sheets for providers to guide deprescribing of several medication classes	• Contains general information on principles as well as specific evidence for and against deprescribing for each class • Algorithm for deprescribing included (based on Scott et al,[44] article on deprescribing) • Medication-specific algorithm in each fact sheet	• Needs more evidence of use in practice or effect on health outcomes
Overuse and underuse	START and STOPP Criteria	Article	O'Mahony D, O'Sullivan D, Byrne S, et al. STOPP/START criteria for potentially inappropriate prescribing in older people: version 2. *Age Ageing* 2015;44(2):213–8.	https://www.ncbi.nlm.nih.gov/pmc/articles/PMC4339726/	If/then indicators for starting medication (34 indicators) or stopping medication (80 indicators) in specific clinical situations	• Relatively stronger content, face, and predictive validity than other tools • Potential use as part of computerized decision support	• Time-consuming to implement without a Web tool or device application

(continued on next page)

Table 3
(continued)

Problem	Tool	Type	Source	Link	Description	Pros	Cons
Overuse and PIM use	MedStopper	Web tool	University of British Columbia, funded by Canadian Institute for Health Information	http://medstopper.com/	Web-based tool in which clinical information and medication list are entered and a ranked list is provided for medications to be reduced or stopped. Rankings were made by a consensus of experts based on a medication's potential to improve symptoms, to reduce the risk of future illness, and likelihood of harm	• Tapering recommendations also given • Incorporates recommendations from Beers Criteria and STOPP Criteria	• Consensus and ranking process unclear and not published in a peer-reviewed publication

PIM use	Beers Criteria	Article	American Geriatrics Society Beers Criteria Update Expert Panel. *J Am Geriatr Soc* 1015;63:2227–46.	http://onlinelibrary.wiley.com/store/10.1111/jgs.13702.pdf?v=1&t=j3aupnid8s=8bf6c9562ef7ebc924588cfc510941afdb12fb3e	Criteria developed by a 13-member expert panel and periodically updated. Contains a list of drugs to avoid, drug-disease combinations to avoid, drugs to use with caution in renal impairment, and drugs with strong anticholinergic properties	• Frequently updated to incorporate current evidence • Renal dosing and anticholinergic lists are relative strengths	• Recommendation is to use in conjunction with other tools, such as the STOPP criteria • Time-consuming to use without Web or computer decision support • Can be searched with a device application that is proprietary ($9.99/year) • Needs more information on alternative medications
Overuse	Polypharmacy Guidance	Web page and device application	National Health Service Scotland	http://www.polypharmacy.scot.nhs.uk/	List of 7 steps for medication review and polypharmacy reduction	• Includes evidence that is updated on efficacy and safety of medications, with data presented in terms of number needed to treat and common adverse drug reactions	• Tool is more implicit and may be difficult to use in a busy encounter

Note: In addition to the tools presented here, several others are available.[45]

that pharmacists can lead is medication reconciliation. After that, pharmacists can conduct a comprehensive medication review to assess for the presence of overuse, PIM use, or underuse. One specific area that pharmacists can reduce medication-related risk among older adults is regarding fall risk. Importantly, the Centers for Disease Control and Prevention and the American Pharmacists Association recently released a free, online, application-based module called The Pharmacist's Role in Older Adult Fall Prevention.[30] Pharmacists can learn how to identify modifiable risk factors, such as medication use, and how to use effective clinical and community strategies to reduce risk.

Challenges and Considerations

General

The process of screening for medication appropriateness in older adults is challenging and time consuming. Although this process can confer tremendous benefits, it is important to recognize the barriers that might arise. Most notably, in the US health care system, clinical information exists in many different, and often disconnected, systems. Simply obtaining an accurate medical problem list and up-to-date medication list is often a rate-limiting step in this process. Unique challenges and considerations to each care setting are now discussed.

Community

In the community setting, older adults often obtain medications from multiple pharmacies. For example, a study of more than 900,000 Medicare Part D beneficiaries found that 38.1% used multiple pharmacies in a single year.[31] Unfortunately, pharmacies from different chains (and sometimes even different pharmacy locations within the same chain) often do not have the capability of real-time data sharing. This lack of data sharing makes obtaining an accurate medication list challenging. In addition, older adults in the community frequently obtain over-the-counter medications and supplements, which are notorious for not being recorded on the older adult's medication list. Several over-the-counter medications may impose a significant risk for older adults (eg, diphenhydramine, aspirin). Comprehensive medication reconciliation is, therefore, critical to safe and effective screening for medication appropriateness in the community.

Hospital

Transitions between the hospital and other care settings are a major challenge because the clinicians caring for the patient in the hospital often have limited information about the patient's medication history. When the patient is discharged from the hospital, information about the medication-related decisions made during the hospital course may not be forwarded to the next care setting. Numerous studies have identified medication discrepancies occurring on hospital discharge.[32–34] Moreover, medication discrepancies are also likely to arise in the hospital setting because the patient's critical illness is given priority; medications are stopped or regimens are modified to help stabilize the patient's acute condition. Furthermore, medication formularies used by hospitals also necessitate medication interchanges and dosage modifications. Clinicians must therefore keep track of a large number of in-hospital medication changes. Even when information regarding medications is available, gaps in communication between the hospital and other settings represent a major barrier.[35,36]

Nursing home

Major barriers to screening for medication appropriateness in the nursing home (NH) are low physician involvement in daily care and high staff turnover.[37,38] Low physician involvement and high staff turnover often translate into limited provider-pharmacist and staff-pharmacist interaction, creating an additional barrier to screening because the pharmacist might not have the necessary information to perform medication appropriateness screening. A lack of connectivity between the NH and other care settings often creates additional communication challenges that prevent meaningful screening. Health care professionals have many competing demands on their time. Literature has shown that when clinicians are faced with multiple competing tasks, one task will often dominate the agenda of a patient encounter, and medication appropriateness screening is often not that dominating task.[39] The high clinical complexity of NH residents, especially after they transition from an acute care setting, places even more demands on the clinician. Finally, there is a significant lack of evidence about the outcomes of medication use for frail older individuals with multiple comorbidities, such as those who reside in the NH setting.[40] The absence of evidence for NH residents undermines clinicians' ability to screen for medication appropriateness by creating uncertainty over whether residents will benefit from prescribing or discontinuation of many treatments.

FUTURE DIRECTIONS TO IMPROVE SCREENING FOR MEDICATION APPROPRIATENESS

Adoption of screening for appropriate medication use in older adults can be viewed as a stepwise process (**Fig. 1**). This process begins with awareness and prioritization, followed by passive and then active screening, and finally full integration. It is important for health care systems to identify their starting point in this process in order to effectively plan their efforts. Two key areas for future directions are development and integration of semiautomated medication appropriateness screening and advancing a US-based national consortium for these efforts.

Semiautomation for Faster Medication Appropriateness Screening

The time and effort required to conduct medication appropriateness screening create a critical need for the development of efficient and innovative approaches and tools.

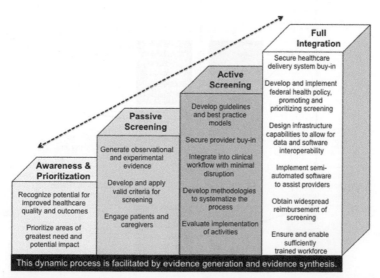

Fig. 1. Adoption of appropriate medication use screening in the elderly. (*Adapted from* IMS Institute for Healthcare Informatics. Patient adoption of mhealth: use, evidence and remaining barriers of mainstream acceptance 2015)

The field of computer science may offer some potentially relevant approaches and techniques. In particular, computer science techniques using semiautomated medication appropriateness screening are promising. Semiautomated medication appropriateness screening would rely on the application of text-mining techniques to the EMR. The application of text mining algorithms to EMR data would help to distinguish the highest priority or most urgent problems from those that are lower priority or nonurgent (**Fig. 2**). After the initial training of the text mining algorithms, little additional effort would be required from the clinician or medical team while the algorithms work in the background as care is provided to patients.

National Efforts

Policymakers, health care institutions, and consortia of researchers and clinicians combining efforts might be the best way to address improvements in medication appropriateness. However, to the best of the authors' knowledge, the US does not currently have such efforts in place. One example is the SIMPATHY Project (Stimulating Innovative Management of Polypharmacy and Adherence in the Elderly). SIMPATHY is a consortium of health care providers, researchers, and policymakers across 10 institutions in several EU countries and led by the Scottish Government. The goal is to promote community-based interventions that will empower patients and provide resources to address appropriate medication use and adherence.[41] Similarly, the SENATOR project (Software ENgine for the Assessment & optimization of

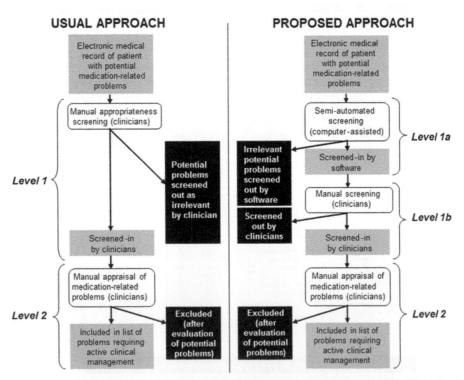

Fig. 2. Potential application of statistical pattern learning algorithms to medication appropriateness screening. (*Courtesy of* Thomas Trikalinos, MD, PhD, Brown University School of Public Health, Providence, RI; adapted with permission.)

drug and non-drug Therapy in Older peRsons) is a multinational consortium of researchers from 12 institutions in the EU that is developing a Web-based platform to improve the appropriateness of pharmacologic as well as nonpharmacologic therapy in older adults.[42] The group is developing a Web-based medication screening tool based on the START/STOPP criteria and is conducting clinical trials using the tool.[42]

STRATEGIES FOR IMPROVING SCREENING FOR MEDICATION APPROPRIATENESS

What can we do to improve screening for medication appropriateness in older adults today in light of the current evidence available? The following are some key strategies that are supported by the literature:

1. *Use a team-based approach to ensure accurate medical problem and medication lists.* A large body of literature points to the many difficulties associated with medication reconciliation across care settings. In order to minimize these challenges, a team-based approach is ideal for collecting, documenting, and communicating medication reconciliation information. Health care settings with access to a pharmacist should leverage their medication expertise.
2. *Eliminate unnecessary medications.* Confirm clinical indications for all medications that a patient is taking; discontinue medications without an indication. Determine the effectiveness of medications for the patient; discontinue medications that are not sufficiently effective. Consider the risk/benefit profile of medications on a routine basis because it may change over time. Focus on commonly used medications that are often overprescribed, have questionable benefit, or have safer alternatives available (eg, PPIs, benzodiazepines, hypnotics).
3. *Identify PIMs and consider dose reduction or discontinuation.* Use up-to-date explicit criteria (eg, Beers Criteria, STOPP) as a starting point. Leverage technology to automate as much of this as possible, using dashboards and computer decision support systems.
4. *Identify conditions that are not being treated.* Look for reasons that medications might not be used (eg, limited life expectancy, patient preferences, unfavorable risk/benefit profile) and document those in the EMR. Common clinical scenarios that are undertreated in older adults include cardiovascular conditions, osteoporosis, and conditions requiring anticoagulation.
5. *Note that some of the most clinically necessary medications can also be high risk in certain older adults.* Although much attention is given to those PIMs listed on explicit criteria such as the Beers Criteria, other medications, such as anticoagulants and glucose-lowering agents, are implicated in the most serious adverse drug events (ie, hospitalization). Avoid focusing solely on those medications listed in explicit criteria for medication appropriateness. Reassess the risk/benefit of these other high-risk medications and relax therapeutic goals (eg, A1c%) as needed.
6. *Pay special attention to high-risk periods, such as following transitions of care.* Older adults transitioning across care settings are at the highest risk for inappropriate medication use and the related negative health outcomes. "Double down" on these screening efforts for older adults who have recently had a transition of care.
7. *Take into account the patients' and caregivers' preferences about medication use.* Attention should be given to understanding patient preferences and goals of care. Only then can patient-specific medication recommendations be made and medication regimen monitoring plans developed and implemented. Shared decision making between the patient and the provider is the goal.

SUMMARY

Older adults are at high risk for inappropriate medication use given their myriad medical conditions and medications. Screening efforts may seem overwhelming, but starting with a focused approach and leveraging a team-based strategy can help practicing clinicians gain initial momentum. Future research is needed to strengthen the evidence base for pharmacotherapy in older adults and to elucidate effective and scalable interventions to improve medication safety.

REFERENCES

1. Newman AB, Cauley JA. The epidemiology of aging. Dordrecht (The Netherlands): Springer; 2012.
2. The American Geriatrics Society Expert Panel Members. Guiding principles for the care of older adults with multimorbidity: an approach for clinicians. J Am Geriatr Soc 2012;60(10):E1–25.
3. DiPiro JT. Pharmacotherapy: a pathophysiologic approach. 10th edition. New York: McGraw-Hill Education; 2017.
4. Patterson SM, Cadogan CA, Kerse N, et al. Interventions to improve the appropriate use of polypharmacy for older people. Cochrane Database Syst Rev 2014;(10):CD008165.
5. Gallagher P, Ryan C, Byrne S, et al. STOPP (Screening Tool of Older Person's prescriptions) and START (Screening Tool to Alert doctors to Right Treatment). Consensus validation. Int J Clin Pharmacol Ther 2008;46(2):72–83.
6. Chang CB, Chan DC. Comparison of published explicit criteria for potentially inappropriate medications in older adults. Drugs Aging 2010;27(12):947–57.
7. Radcliff S, Yue JR, Rocco G, et al. American Geriatrics Society 2015 updated Beers criteria for potentially inappropriate medication use in older adults. J Am Geriatr Soc 2015;63(11):2227–46.
8. Barry PJ, Gallagher P, Ryan C, et al. START (screening tool to alert doctors to the right treatment)–an evidence-based screening tool to detect prescribing omissions in elderly patients. Age Ageing 2007;36(6):632–8.
9. Tjia J, Velten SJ, Parsons C, et al. Studies to reduce unnecessary medication use in frail older adults: a systematic review. Drugs Aging 2013;30(5):285–307.
10. Marcum ZA, Amuan ME, Hanlon JT, et al. Prevalence of unplanned hospitalizations caused by adverse drug reactions in older veterans. J Am Geriatr Soc 2012;60(1):34–41.
11. Fried TR, O'Leary J, Towle V, et al. Health outcomes associated with polypharmacy in community-dwelling older adults: a systematic review. J Am Geriatr Soc 2014;62(12):2261–72.
12. Marcum ZA, Pugh MJ, Amuan ME, et al. Prevalence of potentially preventable unplanned hospitalizations caused by therapeutic failures and adverse drug withdrawal events among older veterans. J Gerontol A Biol Sci Med Sci 2012; 67(8):867–74.
13. Meid AD, Lampert A, Burnett A, et al. The impact of pharmaceutical care interventions for medication underuse in older people: a systematic review and meta-analysis. Br J Clin Pharmacol 2015;80(4):768–76.
14. Ernst FR, Grizzle AJ. Drug-related morbidity and mortality: updating the cost-of-illness model. J Am Pharm Assoc (Wash) 2001;41(2):192–9.
15. Bootman JL, Harrison DL, Cox E. The health care cost of drug-related morbidity and mortality in nursing facilities. Arch Intern Med 1997;157(18): 2089–96.

16. Centers for Medicare and Medicaid Services. Readmissions reduction program (HRRP). 2016. Available at: https://www.cms.gov/medicare/medicare-fee-for-service-payment/acuteinpatientpps/readmissions-reduction-program.html. Accessed May 5, 2017.

17. Zaydfudim V, Dossett LA, Starmer JM, et al. Implementation of a real-time compliance dashboard to help reduce SICU ventilator-associated pneumonia with the ventilator bundle. Arch Surg 2009;144(7):656–62.

18. Anderson D, Zlateva I, Khatri K, et al. Using health information technology to improve adherence to opioid prescribing guidelines in primary care. Clin J Pain 2015;31(6):573–9.

19. Dixon BE, Jabour AM, Phillips EO, et al. An informatics approach to medication adherence assessment and improvement using clinical, billing, and patient-entered data. J Am Med Inform Assoc 2014;21(3):517–21.

20. American College of Clinical Pharmacy, McBane SE, Dopp AL, et al. Collaborative drug therapy management and comprehensive medication management-2015. Pharmacotherapy 2015;35(4):e39–50.

21. Peterson JF, Kripalani S, Danciu I, et al. Electronic surveillance and pharmacist intervention for vulnerable older inpatients on high-risk medication regimens. J Am Geriatr Soc 2014;62(11):2148–52.

22. Meulendijk MC, Spruit MR, Drenth-van Maanen AC, et al. Computerized decision support improves medication review effectiveness: an experiment evaluating the STRIP assistant's usability. Drugs Aging 2015;32(6):495–503.

23. O'Sullivan D, O'Mahony D, O'Connor MN, et al. Prevention of adverse drug reactions in hospitalised older patients using a software-supported structured pharmacist intervention: a cluster randomised controlled trial. Drugs Aging 2016;33(1):63–73.

24. Tamblyn R, Huang A, Perreault R, et al. The medical office of the 21st century (MOXXI): effectiveness of computerized decision-making support in reducing inappropriate prescribing in primary care. CMAJ 2003;169(6):549–56.

25. Yourman L, Concato J, Agostini JV. Use of computer decision support interventions to improve medication prescribing in older adults: a systematic review. Am J Geriatr Pharmacother 2008;6(2):119–29.

26. Grion AM, Gallo U, Tinjala DD, et al. A new computer-based tool to reduce potentially inappropriate prescriptions in hospitalized geriatric patients. Drugs Aging 2016;33(4):267–75.

27. MedStopper Beta. 2017. Available at: http://medstopper.com/. Accessed April 27, 2017.

28. Cassels A. 'Can I stop even one of these pills?' The development of a tool to make deprescribing easier. Eur J Hosp Pharm Sci Pract 2017;24(1):3–4.

29. Lee JK, Slack MK, Martin J, et al. Geriatric patient care by U.S. pharmacists in healthcare teams: systematic review and meta-analyses. J Am Geriatr Soc 2013;61(7):1119–27.

30. Centers for Disease Control and Prevention. STEADI - Older Adult Fall Prevention. 2017. Available at: https://www.cdc.gov/steadi/training.html. Accessed April 27, 2017.

31. Marcum ZA, Driessen J, Thorpe CT, et al. Effect of multiple pharmacy use on medication adherence and drug-drug interactions in older adults with Medicare Part D. J Am Geriatr Soc 2014;62(2):244–52.

32. Boockvar KS, Liu S, Goldstein N, et al. Prescribing discrepancies likely to cause adverse drug events after patient transfer. Qual Saf Health Care 2009;18(1):32–6.

33. Boockvar KS, Carlson LaCorte H, Giambanco V, et al. Medication reconciliation for reducing drug-discrepancy adverse events. Am J Geriatr Pharmacother 2006;4(3):236–43.
34. Boockvar K, Fishman E, Kyriacou CK, et al. Adverse events due to discontinuations in drug use and dose changes in patients transferred between acute and long-term care facilities. Arch Intern Med 2004;164(5):545–50.
35. King BJ, Gilmore-Bykovskyi AL, Roiland RA, et al. The consequences of poor communication during transitions from hospital to skilled nursing facility: a qualitative study. J Am Geriatr Soc 2013;61(7):1095–102.
36. Shah F, Burack O, Boockvar KS. Perceived barriers to communication between hospital and nursing home at time of patient transfer. J Am Med Dir Assoc 2010;11(4):239–45.
37. Shield R, Rosenthal M, Wetle T, et al. Medical staff involvement in nursing homes: development of a conceptual model and research agenda. J Appl Gerontol 2014;33(1):75–96.
38. Stone R, Harahan MF. Improving the long-term care workforce serving older adults. Health Aff 2010;29(1):109–15.
39. Miles RW. Cognitive bias and planning error: nullification of evidence-based medicine in the nursing home. J Am Med Dir Assoc 2010;11(3):194–203.
40. Crystal S, Gaboda D, Lucas J, et al. Assessing medication exposures and outcomes in the frail elderly: assessing research challenges in nursing home pharmacotherapy. Med Care 2010;48(6 Suppl):S23–31.
41. Scottish Government Health and Social Care Directorates. Stimulating innovation management of polypharmacy and adherence in the elderly. 2017. Available at: http://www.simpathy.eu/. Accessed June 10, 2017.
42. SENATOR. Development and clinical trials of a new Software ENgine for the Assessment & optimization of drug and non-drug Therapy in Older peRsons. 2017. Available at: https://www.senator-project.eu/. Accessed June 10, 2017.
43. Tannenbaum C, Martin P, Tamblyn R, et al. Reduction of inappropriate benzodiazepine prescriptions among older adults through direct patient education: the EMPOWER cluster randomized trial. JAMA Intern Med 2014;174(6):890–8.
44. Scott IA, Hilmer SN, Reeve E, et al. Reducing inappropriate polypharmacy: the process of deprescribing. JAMA Intern Med 2015;175(5):827–34.
45. Bulloch MN, Olin JL. Instruments for evaluating medication use and prescribing in older adults. J Am Pharm Assoc (2003) 2014;54(5):530–7.

Screening for Geriatric Syndromes
Falls, Urinary/Fecal Incontinence, and Osteoporosis

Erin M. Smith, MD, Amit A. Shah, MD*

KEYWORDS

- Geriatric syndromes • Screening • Urinary incontinence • Fecal incontinence • Falls
- Osteoporosis

KEY POINTS

- History of falls and fear of falling are clues that should trigger a multifactorial assessment of fall risk and targeted interventions to reduce falls.
- Urinary and fecal incontinence are common and underreported by patients. Simple screening questions, such as, "Do you leak or lose control of urine or stool?" can help trigger more detailed assessments and interventions.
- Screening for osteoporosis is indicated for women over age 65. Intervals for follow-up screenings are controversial and can be dictated based on initial test results and a patient's desire for treatment.
- The benefits of screening for osteoporosis in men are uncertain, but likely screening should be done at least once for men over age 70 or at high risk.
- The Fracture Risk Assessment tool can be used to determine which patients are at high risk and who should have bone mineral density screening.

INTRODUCTION

Given the high prevalence of geriatric syndromes and their typical multifactorial etiology, screening can be a high-yield part of a geriatric assessment or geriatric preventative care visit. Given the multifactorial nature of these syndromes, addressing a positive screening often involves a multipronged approach.[1] This article reviews screening for 3 such syndromes, which significantly affect quality of life and functional status of older patients: falls, incontinence, and osteoporosis.

Disclosure Statement: Both Dr E.M. Smith and Dr A.A. Shah have no relationships with any commercial company that has a direct financial interest in subject matter and have no conflicts of interest.
Department of Internal Medicine, Mayo Clinic, 13400 E. Shea Boulevard, Scottsdale, AZ 85259, USA
* Corresponding author.
E-mail address: Shah.Amit@mayo.edu

SCREENING FOR FALLS

Risk of falling and history of prior falls are important components of the geriatric assessment. In the geriatric population, falling and the fear of falling can have a tremendous effect on quality of life and independence.[2] Falls are a significant source of morbidity and mortality in the older adult. The Centers for Disease Control and Prevention (CDC) reports that in 2014 almost 30% of older adults reported a fall, and deaths in older adults due to falls numbered approximately 27,000.[3] The estimated Medicare cost for falls in 2015 was more than $31 billion.[4]

The etiology of falls in older adults is complex and often a combination of environmental factors and disease processes. Increasing age is itself a risk factor for falls. A 90 year old is up to 4 times more likely to fall than a 60 year old.[5] History of falls is a strong predictor of future falls.[6] Medical conditions with an increased risk of falling include lower extremity osteoarthritis, depression, heart disease, and nocturia.[5,7,8] Medications often associated with increased fall risk are sedating or affect gait and balance.[2]

Given how frequent falls are, how devastating the consequences can be, and the availability of interventions to reduce falling, it seems that there would be high-quality evidence for the benefits of screening for falls and who should be routinely screened for falls. Unfortunately, there is not any 1 screening test that has sufficient evidence to support its widespread use in identifying patients at risk of falling who would benefit from interventions to reduce future risk.[6] There is consensus based on expert opinion that screening for falls and risk of falls should be done, because evidence supports that interventions, such as exercise or physical therapy, have moderate benefit in fall prevention.[9]

In the recommendation statement of the U.S. Preventive Services Task Force (USPSTF) for fall prevention, in-depth screening for all community-dwelling older adults is not recommended due to lack of currently available evidence.[6] The USPSTF states that there may be a role for a multifactorial risk assessment in patients with history of falls and certain comorbid diseases, but that the small net benefit is only seen when this is combined with management of fall prevention.[6] In regard to gait and mobility tools in screening for fall risk, the USPSTF determined that there are no validated tools to predict falls, but that the Timed Up and Go Test and the Functional Reach Test predict fall risk and are practical in the constraints of a primary care office (**Box 1**).[6]

Box 1
Timed Up and Go Test and Functional Reach Test

Timed Up and Go Test

- Patients can use walking aid if needed.
- Patient starts sitting back in a standard arm chair.
- Mark off a line 3 m away on the floor
- Measure the time it takes the patient to stand up from the chair, walk to the line at a normal pace, turn, walk back to the chair, and sit down.
- Various cutpoints are used in research studies, but the CDC recommends greater than 12 seconds as a positive screen for a patient at high risk for falls.

Functional Reach Test

- Assesses a patient's stability by measuring the maximum distance an individual can reach forward while standing in a fixed position.
- Patient stands close to, but not touching a wall, with arm that is closer to the wall at 90° of shoulder flexion (reaching out) with a closed fist next to a ruler on the wall.

- Record the starting position at the third metacarpal head (see image A).
- The patient reaches out as far forward as possible without taking a step.
- The location of the third metacarpal is recorded (see image B).
- The difference between the start and end position is the reach distance.
- Five trials are done: 2 practice trials, followed by 3 test trials, which are averaged to obtain the patient's score.
- A Functional Reach Test score of less than 10 in (25.4 cm) is abnormal, and less than 7 in (17.8 cm) indicates high fall risk and is correlated with ADL limitation.

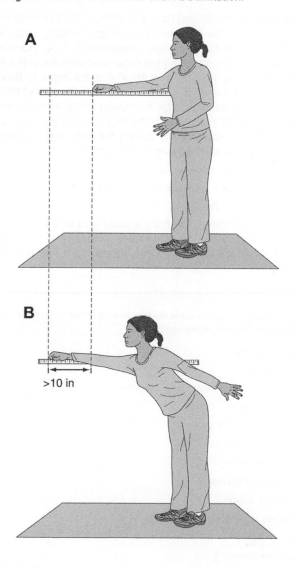

The Functional Reach test.

From Tyner T, Allen DD. Balance and fall risk. In: Cameron MH, Monroe LG, editors. Physical rehabilitation: evidence-based examination, evaluation, and intervention. St Louis (MO): Saunders Elsevier; 2007. p. 320; with permission.

The 2010 Clinical Practice Guideline from the American Geriatrics Society and British Geriatrics Society provides an algorithm for the assessment of fall risk in community dwelling adults over the age of 65.[10] Initial screening for older adults uses questions regarding fall frequency, acute falls, and concerns with gait and balance. Answering yes to any of these questions indicates that a patient is at high risk for falling and would benefit from a more in-depth assessment. This evaluation should include, at minimum, an evaluation of balance and gait and ideally a multifactorial fall risk assessment, which combines screening with intervention plans and identifies modifiable risk factors.

The National Institute for Health and Care Excellence (NICE) provides similar guidelines for adults over age 65 while including screening for osteoporosis and urinary incontinence (UI) in the multifactorial risk assessment.[11] A modified list of the multifactorial risk assessment combining the recommendations of the American Geriatric Society/British Geriatric Society and NICE can be seen in **Box 2**. Screening should be performed at least once a year in adults over the age of 65.[6,11]

In an attempt to make resources for fall screening and prevention available for patients and providers, the CDC has created the Stopping Elderly Accidents, Deaths & Injuries program. The CDC recommends asking the following 3 questions as a part of the routine examination in patients over the age of 65:

1. Have you fallen in the past 12 months?
2. Have you ever felt unsteady with standing or walking?
3. Are you worried about falling?

A "yes" answer to any of these questions should lead to a further assessment. To this end, the CDC has created and made available a fall risk checklist that incorporates the components of the multifactorial fall risk assessment into an easy-to-use and downloadable tool.[12]

Box 2
American Geriatric Society/British Geriatric Society and National Institute for Health and Care Excellence multifactorial fall risk assessment areas

- Comprehensive fall history
- Review of medication list
- Assessment of gait/balance and functional mobility
- Testing of orthostatic vitals
- Evaluation of heart rate and rhythm
- Evaluation of neurologic function
- Evaluation of muscle strength
- Examination of feet and footwear
- Examination of visual acuity
- Assessment of safety home and environment
- Osteoporosis screening
- Urinary incontinence screening

Data from Panel on Prevention of Falls in Older Persons, American Geriatrics Society and British Geriatrics Society. Summary of the Updated American Geriatrics Society/British Geriatrics Society clinical practice guideline for prevention of falls in older persons. J Am Geriatr Soc 2011;59(1):148–57.

Fear of falling is associated with limitations in performing activities of daily living (ADLs), increased risk of future falls, and greater rates of nursing home and assisted living center admissions and, thus, should be included in the fall risk assessment.[13] Although this can be evaluated with a single question, "Do you fear falling?" more detailed assessment tools are available.[13] Examples include the Fall Efficacy Scale and its variations that address an individual's ability to avoid a fall during daily activities or the Activities-specific Balance Confidence Scale that focuses on how balance and steadiness affect ADLs.[14–16] Falling and fear of falling are key medical issues in the older adult that should be a component of the geriatric patient assessment. Asking broad and simple questions initially is an effective tool to determine which patients would benefit from a multifactorial risk assessment and a targeted risk reduction approach.

SCREENING FOR URINARY AND FECAL INCONTINENCE

Urinary and fecal incontinence are common issues experienced by older patients. Compared with younger patients, older adults are less likely to mention incontinence to their providers, reflecting a societal view that incontinence is a normal part of aging.[17] The reluctance to mention incontinence is a key reason why incontinence screening questions should be routinely used in geriatric assessment. The economic and social costs to incontinence are substantial. The financial costs include incontinence care supplies and also increased nursing home admission rates for incontinent patients.[18] Socially, incontinence may cause embarrassment secondary to odor and hygiene and reluctance to leave the home, leading to social isolation and decreased activity levels.[18] Incontinence also carries with it the disruption of sleep and increased risk of falls.[17,19]

Screening for Urinary Incontinence

UI is a complex medical condition defined by the involuntary loss of urine, which can be further divided into 3 main subtypes: stress UI, urgency UI, and mixed UI. Stress UI is more common in women and can be considered a weakness of the urethral sphincter, and symptoms are related to increased pressure due to sneezing and coughing.[20,21] Urgency UI is more common in older patients and is associated with a sensation of urgency and leakage.[20] Other important causes of incontinence include functional UI, associated with decreased will or ability for appropriate toileting, and overflow incontinence.[17]

Evaluating for risk factors is an important component in the assessment of UI in the older adult. In men and women, increased age, genetics, obesity, and tobacco use are associated factors.[17] In women, multiparity is associated with UI. In men, the term, *lower urinary tract symptoms*, includes changes in urine storage and voiding that may be due to prostate pathology, with other etiologies also deserving attention.[22] Conservative and invasive therapeutic options are available for the older adult with UI. Because of the social and economic costs of incontinence and, in many cases, the availability of effective therapeutic options, it is important for providers to assess the need for intervention or specialist referral.

There are many questionnaires used as screening tools that are practical in the primary setting. For use in primary care, the authors recommend the 3 Incontinence Questions questionnaire, which is brief and has good sensitivity and specificity. Specifically, it asks patients about the presence of incontinence and activities associated with urine leakage to differentiate between stress UI and urgency UI.[23] Once incontinence is identified, 2 important roles of screening should be to determine whether symptoms represent an acute or chronic process and whether a patient can be managed conservatively or surgically. Causes of transient UI, including infection, constipation, change in functional status, and medications, must be addressed for new-onset or acutely worsening incontinence.[20] Complicated incontinence, which includes multiple infections, hematuria, severe voiding difficulties, prior pelvic radiation, prior surgery, fistula, and, in women, significant uterine prolapse, needs to be referred to a specialist because procedures, such as cystoscopy or urodynamic testing, or surgical treatments may be indicated.[24]

Various societies have produced guidelines for the screening and management of UI. The American College of Physicians, American College of Obstetricians and Gynecologists, and the American Urogynecologic Society make specific emphasis that because patients underreport their symptoms, providers should intentionally ask about symptoms of UI.[25,26] Physicians should perform a thorough history and physical examination as part of the assessment of UI, with focus on differentiating between stress UI, urgency UI, and mixed UI.[21,26,27] The history should assess acuity of symptom onset and frequency of symptoms.[26] Surgical society guidelines emphasize using questionnaires to assess level of bother and quality of life more than other groups and this likely reflects the need to assess whether a patient is willing and capable of undergoing a surgical procedure.[22,24,28,29] A screening physical examination typically includes a general, abdominal, pelvic, rectal, and neurologic evaluation.[22,24,25,27] A cough stress examination may also be indicated when there is high suspicion for stress UI and is considered positive if fluid is visualized at the urethra after coughing with a full bladder.[25,29]

Most experts recommend testing urinalysis in patients with new or worsening incontinence symptoms to assess for infection.[24,25,27,29] In men, measurement of renal function may be indicated in patients with urinary retention or suspicion for hydronephrosis and obstructive uropathy causing renal impairment.[22] Completion of a bladder diary, evaluation of urethral mobility, and obtaining urodynamic studies have a role in the assessment of UI rather than screening.[21,25,27,29,30] Similarly, the measuring of postvoid residuals is generally not incorporated into screening for UI but may be useful in diagnosis or determining a treatment plan.[24,25] Urodynamic studies, measure of urethral function, electromyography, and cystometry are not needed in the initial evaluation, and treatment can often be started without these additional studies.[25,30]

Screening for Fecal Incontinence

Although less common than UI, fecal incontinence is also seen with advancing age. Studies show that fecal incontinence can affect up to 15% of people over the age of 70, but that fewer than 30% of patients discuss this problem with their provider.[31] Defined as the unintentional loss of stool, fecal incontinence can have a significant impact on socialization and quality of life, including being a key factor in assisted living or nursing home placement and an important component to consider in decreasing skin breakdown and risk for pressure-induced skin injuries.[32,33] A common cause of fecal incontinence in older patients is actually constipation causing fecal retention and fecal impaction. This fecal impaction disrupts the internal anal sphincter tone and results in leakage of stool around the impaction. Studies have shown a great deal of underdiagnosis and underreporting of fecal incontinence, with 1 study showing only 2.7% of patients with fecal incontinence carried that diagnosis in their medical records.[34] There are no validated questionnaires used for screening for fecal incontinence in the primary care setting, and the authors recommend use of the following simple question, "Do you ever leak or lose control of stool (your bowels)?"

Certain risk factors that may indicate a need for screening are constipation, the need to manually disimpact stool to have a bowel movement, diarrhea, increased age, increased body mass index, chronic diseases, history of irritable bowel syndrome, history of inflammatory bowel disease, history of cholecystectomy, and history of vaginal delivery.[32] A complete physical examination should include visual inspection of the rectum, digital rectal examination, and anoscopy.[35] In the absence of alarm symptoms (weight loss, hematochezia, abdominal mass, or neurologic deficits) and need for urgent referral, fecal incontinence may be managed medically with treatments, including dietary modification, stool-bulking agents, and bowel training.[24,36] The American College of Gastroenterology does not recommend any further testing as part of the initial assessment unless a patient does not respond to conservative treatment.[32] Further testing can be done if there is no response, including flexible sigmoidoscopy, colonoscopy, barium enema, anorectal manometry, balloon expulsion test, defecography, pudendal nerve terminal latencies, anal endosonography, and endoanal MRI, typically under the guidance of a gastroenterologist or colorectal surgeon.[36] Specialized nonsurgical and nonmedication treatments, such as biofeedback and pelvic floor physical therapy, are often underutilized and with good evidence of effectiveness and should be pursued for patients who have at least some preserved voluntary sphincter contraction.[36]

In summary, urinary and fecal incontinence are common problems. Simple screening questions, such as "Do you leak or lose control of urine or stool?" should be a part of all geriatric assessments. If positive, more detailed questions should be asked to identify patients who would benefit from behavioral, biofeedback, medication, or surgical interventions that can help improve quality of life and reduce morbidity for the older patient.

SCREENING FOR OSTEOPOROSIS

Osteoporosis is the change in bone structure and density, which increases the risk of fragility fractures in adults even in the absence of falls.[37] These fractures can lead to hospitalization, loss of independence, chronic pain, and debility.[38–40] Although women are at increased risk of osteoporosis due to estrogen deprivation with menopause, senile osteoporosis affects men and women and is reflected in the growing incidence of osteoporosis with increased age.[41] In men and women over the age of 80, the rates of osteoporosis are 46.3% and 77.1%, respectively, and 25% of osteoporosis fractures in the United States occur in men.[40,41]

The goal of screening for osteoporosis in the older adult is to determine which individuals would benefit from therapy to prevent further disease and fragility fractures. This should be measured against the risks of screening, which include radiation exposure, costs, time, and side effects of potential therapeutic interventions, and whether a patient will live long enough to benefit from these medications.[42]

Various professional societies have produced guidelines for the screening of osteoporosis, which reflects both the scope and complexity of osteoporosis and fragility fractures in the population. A summary of society recommendations for the screening for osteoporosis in men and women is provided in **Table 1**. Although these guidelines present similar recommendations for women over the age of 65, variability is most noticeable in determining the interval of screening and in recommendations for screening in men. Because screening is performed with an intention to treat, clinicians should be familiar with the following recommendations while using an individualized approach with each patient.

Table 1
Summary of recommendations for osteoporosis screening from various national and international organizations

	U.S. Preventive Services Task Force (2011)[43]	American College of Physicians (2008 and 2017) Guidelines[45,48]	National Osteoporosis Foundation (2014)[42]	International Society for Clinical Densitometry (2015)[47]	The American College of Obstetricians and Gynecologists (2012)[44]	Endocrine Society Guideline for Osteoporosis in Men (2012)[46]
Women	Screen all women ≥ age 65 with no upper limit to stop screening. Women < age 65 with fracture risk calculated as ≥ a 65-year-old white woman with no other risk factors	All women ≥ age 65 after a discussion of patient preferences, fracture risk profile, and benefits, harms, and costs of medications	All women ≥ age 65. All women with any fracture age ≥50. Postmenopausal women with other risk factors for fracture	All women ≥ age 65. Postmenopausal women age 50–65 when risk factors are present	Screen all women > age 65	N/A (this guideline covers men only)
Men	Insufficient evidence to make a recommendation for screening in men	Assess all older men for risk factors of osteoporosis (No exact age reported) Screen all men using DXA who have increased osteoporosis risk and are willing to be treated	Screen all men ≥ age 70. All men with any fracture age ≥50. Men age 50–69 with other risk factors for fractures	All men ≥ age 70. Men age 50–70 when risk factors are present	N/A (this guideline covers women only)	Screen all men ≥ age 70. Screen all older men with risk factors of osteoporosis. Screen all men who have had fractures after age 50

Screening interval	Optimal interval is uncertain	Do not screen frequently women with normal bone density because women with normal DXA scores did not progress to osteoporosis within 15 y.	Retesting 1–2 y after initiating medical therapy for osteoporosis and every 2 y thereafter	Intervals between bone mineral density testing should be individualized. Typically, 1 year after therapy change and then with longer intervals once therapeutic effect is established. In patients at risk for rapid bone loss, such as glucocorticoid therapy, testing should be done more frequently.	Screening intervals: • T-score > −1.5: Every 15 y • T-score −1.5 to −1.99: Every 5 y • T-score −2.0 to −2.49: Yearly assessment Use with FRAX tool each year to assess for high risk for fracture for all	Not specified
Other comments	Screening tool should be DXA, with best evidence for the lumbar spine and hip	Do not monitor bone mineral density during the initial 5 y of treatment in patients receiving pharmacologic agents to treat osteoporosis	Risk factors for fractures: includes the risk factors incorporated into FRAX, fall risk, and use of medications known to cause osteoporosis, such as glucocorticoids in a daily dose ≥5 mg prednisone or equivalent for ≥3 mo	DXA is the preferred method for screening and determining therapy	Risk factors that may indicate earlier screening: history of fragility fracture, family history of hip fracture, weight <127 pounds, medications or conditions associated with bone loss, tobacco and/or alcohol use, rheumatoid arthritis	Measure forearm DXA when spine or hip bone mineral density cannot be interpreted and for men with hyperparathyroidism or receiving androgen-deprivation therapy for prostate cancer

In general, it is recommended that all women over the age of 65 should be screened for osteoporosis with dual-energy x-ray absorptiometry (DXA) of the lumbar spine and hip.[43] Postmenopausal women less than 65 years of age and older men should be assessed for risk factors of osteoporosis to determine who should undergo DXA testing.[42–47] The Fracture Risk Assessment (FRAX) tool is available free of charge (https://www.sheffield.ac.uk/FRAX/index.aspx) and can be used to prognosticate a 10-year fracture risk for an individual patient and make decisions for further screening.[42–44] The National Osteoporosis Foundation, Endocrine Society, and International Society for Clinical Densitometry recommend screening for all men over the age of 70.[42,46,47]

SUMMARY

In conclusion, treatment of the older adult is complex, and many conditions pertinent to this age group are multifactorial. This interrelationship is an integral component to the approach to geriatric syndromes, which should be screened for because there are effective interventions available. Fracture-related injury can be devastating in the older adult, and it may reflect a combination of fall risk and osteoporosis. Screening for falls and incontinence can be as simple as asking a few questions, with more detailed assessments used to address prevention or treatment options. Specific recommendations are available for the screening of these conditions and should serve as a guide for the provider in the care of the geriatric population.

REFERENCES

1. Carlson C, Merel SE, Yukawa M. Geriatric syndromes and geriatric assessment for the generalist. Med Clin North Am 2015;99(2):263–79.
2. Phelan EA, Mahoney JE, Voit JC, et al. Assessment and management of fall risk in primary care settings. Med Clin North Am 2015;99(2):281–93.
3. Bergen G, Stevens MR, Burns ER. Falls and fall injuries among adults aged ≥65 years — United States, 2014. MMWR Morb Mortal Wkly Rep 2016;65:993–8. Available at: https://www.cdc.gov/mmwr/volumes/65/wr/mm6537a2.htm?s_cid=mm6537a2_w. Accessed May 25, 2017.
4. Centers for Disease Control and Prevention. Costs of falls among older adults. Available at: https://www.cdc.gov/HomeandRecreationalSafety/Falls/fallcost.html. Accessed May 25, 2017.
5. Stenhagen M, Ekstrom H, Nordell E, et al. Falls in the general elderly population: a 3- and 6- year prospective study of risk factors using data from the longitudinal population study 'Good ageing in Skane'. BMC Geriatr 2013;13:81.
6. Moyer VA. Prevention of falls in community-dwelling older adults: U.S. Preventive Services Task Force recommendation statement. Ann Intern Med 2012;157(3):197–204.
7. Iaboni A, Flint AJ. The complex interplay of depression and falls in older adults: a clinical review. Am J Geriatr Psychiatry 2013;21(5):484–92.
8. Zasadzka E, Borowicz AM, Roszak M, et al. Assessment of the risk of falling with the use of timed up and go test in the elderly with lower extremity osteoarthritis. Clin Interv Aging 2015;10:1289–98.
9. Gillespie LD, Robertson MC, Gillespie WJ, et al. Interventions for preventing falls in older people living in the community. Cochrane Database Syst Rev 2012;(9):CD007146.
10. Panel on Prevention of Falls in Older Persons, American Geriatrics Society and British Geriatrics Society. Summary of the Updated American Geriatrics

Society/British Geriatrics Society clinical practice guideline for prevention of falls in older persons. J Am Geriatr Soc 2011;59(1):148–57.

11. National Institute for Health and Care Excellence. Falls in older people: assessing risk and prevention. Clinical guideline. 2013. Available at: https://www.nice.org.uk/guidance/cg161. Accessed May 25, 2017.

12. STEADI- Older Adult Fall Prevention. 2017. Available at: https://www.cdc.gov/steadi/index.html. Accessed May 25, 2017.

13. Cumming RG, Salkeld G, Thomas M, et al. Prospective study of the impact of fear of falling on activities of daily living, SF-36 scores, and nursing home admission. J Gerontol A Biol Sci Med Sci 2000;55(5):M299–305.

14. Jorstad EC, Hauer K, Becker C, et al. Measuring the psychological outcomes of falling: a systematic review. J Am Geriatr Soc 2005;53(3):501–10.

15. Powell LE, Myers AM. The Activities-specific balance confidence (ABC) Scale. J Gerontol A Biol Sci Med Sci 1995;50A(1):M28–34.

16. Tinetti ME, Richman D, Powell L. Falls efficacy as a measure of fear of falling. J Gerontol 1990;45(6):P239–43.

17. Gibson W, Wagg A. New horizons: urinary incontinence in older people. Age Ageing 2014;43(2):157–63.

18. Milsom I, Coyne KS, Nicholson S, et al. Global prevalence and economic burden of urgency urinary incontinence: a systematic review. Eur Urol 2014;65(1):79–95.

19. Stenzelius K, Molander U, Odeberg J, et al. The effect of conservative treatment of urinary incontinence among older and frail older people: a systematic review. Age Ageing 2015;44(5):736–44.

20. Parker WP, Griebling TL. Nonsurgical Treatment of urinary incontinence in elderly women. Clin Geriatr Med 2015;31(4):471–85.

21. Seehusen DA. Treatments for urinary incontinence in women. Am Fam Physician 2013;87(10):726–8.

22. Gratzke C, Bachmann A, Descazeaud A, et al. EAU guidelines on the assessment of non-neurogenic male lower urinary tract symptoms including benign prostatic obstruction. Eur Urol 2015;67(6):1099–109.

23. Brown JS, Bradley CS, Subak LL, et al. The sensitivity and specificity of a simple test to distinguish between urge and stress urinary incontinence. Ann Intern Med 2006;144(10):715–23.

24. Abrams P, Andersson KE, Birder L, et al. Fourth International Consultation on incontinence recommendations of the International Scientific Committee: evaluation and treatment of urinary incontinence, pelvic organ prolapse, and fecal incontinence. Neurourol Urodyn 2010;29(1):213–40.

25. Committee on Practice Bulletins—Gynecology and the American Urogynecologic Society. ACOG practice bulletin no. 155: urinary incontinence in women. Obstet Gynecol 2015;126(5):e66–81.

26. Qaseem A, Dallas P, Forciea MA, et al. Nonsurgical management of urinary incontinence in women: a clinical practice guideline from the American College of Physicians. Ann Intern Med 2014;161(6):429–40.

27. Burkhard FC, Bosch JLHR, Cruz F, et al. Urinary incontinence. European association of urology non-oncology guidelines 2017. Available at: http://uroweb.org/guideline/urinary-incontinence/. Accessed May 25, 2017.

28. Abrams P, Chapple C, Khoury S, et al. Evaluation and treatment of lower urinary tract symptoms in older men. J Urol 2013;189(1 Suppl):S93–101.

29. Kobashi KC, Albo ME, Dmochowski RR, et al. Surgical treatment of female stress urinary incontinence (SUI): AUA/SUFU Guideline. Clinical Guidelines 2017.

Available at: http://www.auanet.org/guidelines/stress-urinary-incontinence-(sui)-new-(aua/sufu-guideline-2017). Accessed May 11, 2017.

30. Collins CW, Winters JC, American Urological Association, Society of Urodynamics Female Pelvic Medicine and Urogenital Reconstruction. AUA/SUFU adult urodynamics guideline: a clinical review. Urol Clin North Am 2014;41(3):353–62, vii.

31. Kunduru L, Kim SM, Heymen S, et al. Factors that affect consultation and screening for fecal incontinence. Clin Gastroenterol Hepatol 2015;13(4):709–16.

32. Wald A, Bharucha AE, Cosman BC, et al. ACG clinical guideline: management of benign anorectal disorders. Am J Gastroenterol 2014;109(8): 1141–57 [quiz: 1058].

33. Landefeld CS, Bowers BJ, Feld AD, et al. National Institutes of Health state-of-the-science conference statement: prevention of fecal and urinary incontinence in adults. Ann Intern Med 2008;148(6):449–58.

34. Dunivan GC, Heymen S, Palsson OS, et al. Fecal incontinence in primary care: prevalence, diagnosis, and health care utilization. Am J Obstet Gynecol 2010; 202(5):493.e1-6.

35. Fargo MV, Latimer KM. Evaluation and management of common anorectal conditions. Am Fam Physician 2012;85(6):624–30.

36. Paquette IM, Varma MG, Kaiser AM, et al. The American Society of Colon and Rectal Surgeons' clinical practice guideline for the treatment of fecal incontinence. Dis Colon Rectum 2015;58(7):623–36.

37. Duque G, Troen BR. Understanding the mechanisms of senile osteoporosis: new facts for a major geriatric syndrome. J Am Geriatr Soc 2008;56(5):935–41.

38. Singer A, Exuzides A, Spangler L, et al. Burden of illness for osteoporotic fractures compared with other serious diseases among postmenopausal women in the United States. Mayo Clin Proc 2015;90(1):53–62.

39. Baczyk G, Samborski W, Jaracz K. Evaluation of the quality of life of postmenopausal osteoporotic and osteopenic women with or without fractures. Arch Med Sci 2016;12(4):819–27.

40. Burge R, Dawson-Hughes B, Solomon DH, et al. Incidence and economic burden of osteoporosis-related fractures in the United States, 2005-2025. J Bone Miner Res 2007;22(3):465–75.

41. Wright NC, Saag KG, Dawson-Hughes B, et al. The impact of the new National Bone Health Alliance (NBHA) diagnostic criteria on the prevalence of osteoporosis in the USA. Osteoporos Int 2017;28(4):1225–32.

42. Cosman F, de Beur SJ, LeBoff MS, et al. Clinician's Guide to prevention and treatment of osteoporosis. Osteoporos Int 2014;25(10):2359–81.

43. U. S. Preventive Services Task Force. Screening for osteoporosis: U.S. preventive services task force recommendation statement. Ann Intern Med 2011;154(5): 356–64.

44. Committee on Practice Bulletins-Gynecology, The American College of Obstetricians and Gynecologists. ACOG Practice Bulletin N. 129. Osteoporosis. Obstet Gynecol 2012;120(3):718–34.

45. Qaseem A, Snow V, Shekelle P, et al. Screening for osteoporosis in men: a clinical practice guideline from the American College of Physicians. Ann Intern Med 2008;148(9):680–4.

46. Watts NB, Adler RA, Bilezikian JP, et al. Osteoporosis in men: an Endocrine Society clinical practice guideline. J Clin Endocrinol Metab 2012;97(6):1802–22.

47. 2015 ISCD Official Positions – Adult. Available at: http://www.iscd.org/official-positions/2015-iscd-official-positions-adult/. Accessed May 2, 2017.

48. Qaseem A, Forciea MA, McLean RM, et al, Clinical Guidelines Committee of the American College of Physicians. Treatment of low bone density or osteoporosis to prevent fractures in men and women: a clinical practice guideline update from the American College of Physicians. Ann Intern Med 2017;166(11):818–39.

Screening Older Adults for Mental Disorders

Gary J. Kennedy, MD[a],*, Mirnova E. Ceïde, MD[a,b,c]

KEYWORDS

- Aging • Depression • Anxiety • Cognitive impairment

KEY POINTS

- Depression, anxiety, and cognitive impairment are prevalent among older adults, but often go unrecognized, which reduces the patient's independence and burdens the family.
- Interventions to reduce associated costs, morbidity, and mortality, make screening for depression, anxiety, and cognitive impairment imperative.
- Nonetheless, even brief screening procedures for common mental disorders conducted without linking them to accessible interventions will overburden providers and demoralize patients.
- Evidence supporting screening and treatment models for depression in primary care is compelling and portrays the steps necessary to demonstrate the utility of screening for anxiety and cognitive impairment.

INTRODUCTION

A burdensome screening process, like a burdensome intervention, may be challenging for health care providers to perform and for patients to accept. Thus, screening instruments need to be chosen for ease of administration and alignment with intervention.[1] Consequently, the US Preventive Services Task Force (USPSTF) has graded depression screening with B recommendation (moderate benefit) but stipulates that depression care supports must be in place to assure treatment and follow-up.[2]

Disclosure: Dr G.J. Kennedy receives royalties from *The Guilford Press* for *Geriatric Depression: A Clinical Guide*.
[a] Division of Geriatric Psychiatry, Department of Psychiatry and Behavioral Science, Montefiore Medical Center, Albert Einstein College of Medicine, 111 East 210th Street, Bronx, NY 10467, USA; [b] Division of Geriatric Medicine, Department of Psychiatry and Behavioral Science, Montefiore Medical Center, Albert Einstein College of Medicine, 111 East 210th Street, Bronx, NY 10467, USA; [c] Department of Internal Medicine, Montefiore Medical Center, Albert Einstein College of Medicine, 111 East 210th Street, Bronx, NY 10467, USA
* Corresponding author.
E-mail address: gkennedy@montefiore.org

Clin Geriatr Med 34 (2018) 69–79
https://doi.org/10.1016/j.cger.2017.09.005
0749-0690/18/© 2017 Elsevier Inc. All rights reserved.

Incentives

With the transformation of the fee-for-service model of health care financing, primary care is expected to minimize care costs by reducing testing, emergency visits, hospitalizations, and lengths of stay in nursing and rehabilitation facilities. Chronic obstructive pulmonary disease, congestive heart failure, type 2 diabetes, back pain, and arthritis are conditions with costs that are thought to be the most modifiable.[3] Depression increases the morbidity and mortality of these conditions, and depression care decreases both.[4] As the prevalence of impaired cognition increases, screening older adults to prolong their independence is critical for health care financing as well.[5]

During the Medicare Part B Annual Wellness Visit,[6] the provider collects information on psychosocial risks, behavioral risks, and instrumental activities of daily living. Required elements for reimbursement include screening for depression and the assessment of cognitive function. A screening instrument is not required for cognitive impairment as it is for depression. Providers are expected to counsel beneficiaries on interventions.[6] Depression screening can also be billed as code G0444, provided a depression care team is available for interventions. There is also a care planning code G0505 for individuals with impaired cognition.[7,8] This code, which is defined as moderate to high complexity, provides a financial incentive to detect impaired cognition.

DEPRESSION

Primary care practices that integrate a depression care manager can reduce mortality rates among depressed patients with high multimorbidity scores to the level of those with low scores.[9] Depression is a substantial and independent predictor of all-cause mortality among patients with heart failure. Although, antidepressant therapy has not been shown to improve survival or improved cardiovascular status,[10] cognitive behavioral therapy has been associated with reduced anxiety, fatigue, improved social functioning, and quality of life.[10]

Instruments

There are well-established depression screens.[11–14] However, the 9-item Patient Health Questionnaire (PHQ)-9 is more commonly used in primary care settings. At a score of 10 or greater, the PHQ-9 reaches a sensitivity of 88% and specificity of 88% for major depression.[15] **Table 1** displays the PHQ-9 items that match the *Diagnostic and Statistical Manual of Mental Disorders*, 5th edition (DSM-5)[16] depressive symptoms. Either depressed mood or loss of interest and pleasure must be present most days in last 2 weeks and be socially debilitating. These first 2 questions make up the 2-item PHQ[17] and is included in the Centers for Disease Control online sample Health Risk Assessments of the Annual Wellness Assessment.[18] A PHQ-2 score of 3 or greater requires that the PHQ-9 be completed, which can then be used as an indicator for the initiation of treatment or psychiatric consultation (**Table 2**).

The PHQ-9 may be administered by phone without sacrificing validity.[19,20] Telephone administration may be less embarrassing for the patient[21] and more effective at reducing mental health disparities among disadvantaged minority groups.[22] Serial administration of the PHQ-9 can be used to determine treatment responsiveness as well[23] (**Table 3**).

ANXIETY

The prevalence of anxiety disorders among community dwelling older adults is higher than the general population, 11.6% versus 7%, respectively, and associated with

Table 1
The 9-item Patient Health Questionnaire screening questions and complete assessment

Two Question Screening with the PHQ-2				
Over the Last 2 wk, How Often Have You Been Bothered by the Following Problems?	Not at All	Several Days	More Than Half the Days	Nearly Every Day
A. Little interest or pleasure in doing things?	0	1	2	3
B. Feeling down, depressed, or hopeless?	0	1	2	3

If A and B Total 3 or More, Ask the Following:				
Over the Last 2 wk, How Often Have You Been Bothered by the Following Problems?	Not at All	Several Days	More Than Half the Days	Nearly Every Day
Feeling tired or having little energy?	0	1	2	3
Poor appetite or overeating?	0	1	2	3
Trouble falling or staying asleep, or sleeping too much?	0	1	2	3
Feeling bad about yourself, or that you are a failure or have let yourself or your family down?	0	1	2	3
Trouble concentrating on things, such as reading the newspaper or watching television?	0	1	2	3
Moving or speaking so slowly that other people could have noticed? Or the opposite, being so fidgety or restless that you have been moving around a lot more than usual?	0	1	2	3
Thoughts that you would be better off dead or of hurting yourself?	0	1	2	3
Have your feelings caused you distress or interfered with your ability to get along socially with family or friends?	0	1	2	3

Additional information available at: http://phqscreeners.com. Accessed October 9, 2017.

increased mortality in older men.[24] Life-long anxiety symptoms may be mistaken for personality traits rather than a treatable disorder.[25] Certain populations are at elevated risk for anxiety, including those with advanced macular degeneration[26] and medically ill patients.[27] Older women are more likely to develop anxiety disorders in late life than men.[28] The identification of anxiety in older adults using a validated screen is

Table 2
Indications for the initiation of antidepressant treatment based on the 9-item Patient Health Questionnaire

PHQ-9 Score	Depression Severity	Clinician Response
1–4	None	None
5–9	Mild to moderate	If not currently treated, rescreen in 2 wk If currently treated, optimize antidepressant and rescreen in 2 wk
10–15	Major depressive disorder	Initiate antidepressant
≥15	Major depressive disorder	Initiate antidepressant Obtain psychiatric consultation if suicidality or psychosis suspected

Table 3
Prescriber response guidelines at 4 weeks based on the Patient Health Questionnaire and the Sequenced Treatment Alternatives to Relieve Depression (STAR*D) studies

PHQ-9 Score or Change	Outcome	Clinician Response
No decrease or increase	Nonresponse	Switch medication
2–4 points decrease	Partial response	Add medication
≥5 point decrease	Response	Maintain medication
PHQ-9 <5	Remission	Maintain medication

Data from Trivedi MH, Fava M, Wisniewski SR, et al. Medication augmentation after the failure of SSRIs for depression. N Engl J Med 2006;354:1243–52.

recommended, particularly in primary care and hospital settings. Unfortunately, the detail of provider responses indicated by the initial and subsequent PHQ-9 scores has yet to emerge for the commonly used anxiety screening instruments offered in **Box 1** and **Table 4**.

Instruments

The Generalized Anxiety Disorder (GAD)-7 is a 7-item self-report questionnaire used in primary care settings. The internal correlation of the GAD-7 is 0.92 and the test-retest reliability was 0.83 (1-week interval).[29] Each question examines the frequency of anxiety symptoms on a scale from 0 (not at all) to 3 (nearly every day). A cutoff score of 5 yields a sensitivity of 70.9% and specificity of 56.8% for any anxiety disorder.[30] A score of 10 or more is considered moderate to severe. Diagnostic specificity is higher for GAD and may be less for disorders such as social anxiety disorder or panic disorder.[29] The first 2 questions of the GAD-7, the GAD-2, are also valid for identifying anxiety disorders in older adults.[31] A total score of 2, which is "several days" for both questions or "more than half the days" for 1 question, on the GAD-2 suggests an anxiety disorder may be present. One item from the GAD-2, "not able to stop worrying or control your worrying," is included as the anxiety screen in the Sample Health Risk Assessment suggested as part of the Annual Wellness Visit.[6]

COGNITIVE IMPAIRMENT

DSM-5[16] identifies 6 cognitive domains that may be impaired and meet criteria for a major neurocognitive disorder (dementia). They include[1] complex attention,[2] executive

Box 1
Single-question anxiety screen taken from the GAD-7 scale and incorporated into the Sample Risk Assessment as part of the Annual Wellness Visit

A response of "most of the time" or "almost all the time" suggests the need to follow through with the full GAD-7.

In the past 2 weeks, how often were you not able to stop worrying or control your worrying?
    Almost all of the time
    Most of the time
    Some of the time
    Almost never

Data from Goetzel RZ, Staley P, Ogden L, et al. A framework for patient-centered health risk assessments – providing health promotion and disease prevention services to Medicare beneficiaries. Available at: http://www.cdc.gov/policy/hst/hra/FrameworkForHRA.pdf. Accessed October 9, 2017.

Table 4
Generalized Anxiety Disorder, 2-item and 7-item scales, self-reporting format

A score of 2 or greater on 1 the first 2 questions (GAD-2) or a score of 5 from all 7 questions (GAD-7) is a validated predictor of an anxiety disorder. A score of 10 or greater represents moderate to severe anxiety.

Over the last 2 weeks, how often have you been bothered by the following problems?

0 (not at all) 1 (several days) 2 (more than half the days) 3 (nearly every day)

1. Feeling nervous, anxious, or on edge	0	1	2	3
2. Not being able to stop or control worrying	0	1	2	3
3. Worrying too much about different things	0	1	2	3
4. Trouble relaxing	0	1	2	3
5. Being so restless that it's hard to sit still	0	1	2	3
6. Becoming easily annoyed or irritable	0	1	2	3
7. Feeling afraid as if something awful might happen	0	1	2	3

Total score (add your column scores) =

If you checked off any problems, how difficult have these made it for you to do your work, take care of things at home, or get along with other people?

Not difficult at all _____

Somewhat difficult _____

Very difficult _____

Extremely difficult _____

Adapted from Wild B, Eckl A, Herzog W, et al. Assessing generalized anxiety disorder in elderly people using the GAD-7 and GAD-2 scales: results of a validation study. Am J Geriatr Psychiatry 2014;22:1029–38; with permission.

Box 2
General instructions when screening for cognitive impairment

- Ask permission by saying "illness and medications can sometimes interfere with memory; could we spend 5 minutes to test your memory?"
- Reward the person's effort ("good, keep going") and withhold identification of errors until end of the examination.
- When presenting words to be remembered verbally without the written list, pause between each and never couple the words with "and."

---

function,[3] learning and memory,[4] language,[5] perceptual motor (gnosis and praxis), and social cognition[6] (awareness of the emotions and states of mind of others). Screening for recent onset of impaired attention, the most salient feature of delirium, is most often done with the Confusion Assessment Method.[32] When attention is impaired other cognitive domains will seem impaired, hence the need to insure that reversible causes are excluded before dementia is diagnosed. Currently, the USPSTF makes no recommendation about universal screening for cognitive impairment due to insufficient evidence on relative benefits and harms of screening.[33] However, patients with signs or symptoms of cognitive impairment may benefit from screening in terms of safety, planning, and other domains.

Instruments

The Saint Louis University Mental Status (SLUMS),[34] the Montreal Cognitive Assessment (MoCA),[35] the Mini-Cog,[36] and the Mini-Mental Status Examination (MMSE)[37]

Box 3
Telephone version of the Memory Impairment Screen

"Please repeat the following 2 words: penny [pause] plate." (Wait for reply.)

"Now, repeat them again please. Which word was money?" (Wait for reply.)

"Which word was a dish?" (Wait for reply.)

"Now repeat the following 2 words: apple [pause] table." (Wait for reply.)

"Repeat them again please." (Wait for reply.)

"Which word represents fruit?" (Wait for reply.)

"Which word represents furniture?" (Wait for reply.)

"We'll return to the words shortly but, first, please count from 1 to 26." (Wait for reply.)

"Please recite the alphabet from A to Z." (Wait for reply.)

"I am going to start a sequence of numbers and letters, when I stop I want you to continue. I-A, 2-B, 3-C, what comes next?" (Wait for reply.)

"Keep going." (Wait for reply.)

"Now, can you recall the first 2 words I asked you to repeat?" (Wait no more than 30 seconds before providing the category cue and score as above.)

"What were the next 2 words I asked you to repeat?" (Wait no more than 30 seconds before providing the category cue and score as in **Table 4**.)

From Lipton RB, Katz MJ, Kuslansky G, et al. Screening for dementia by telephone using the memory impairment screen. J Am Geriatr Soc 2003;51:1382–90; with permission.

Table 5
Memory impairment screen

The patient is shown the table with 4 words and asked to read them each aloud and to remember. The examiner then asks the patient to identify the word associated with a categorical cue. For example, the correct response to the categorical cue "money" is "penny." After all 4 of the cues and responses are complete, an interference task, such as the Oral Trail Making Test part B, is administered for 2 minutes before asking for recall of the 4 words. Words freely recalled count for a score of 2, those requiring the cue for recall count as 1. A score of 5 is questionably normal. A score of 4 is considered impaired.

"Here's a list of words to remember"	"Which word represents a...?"	"We'll return to the words shortly but first..."	"Please tell me the words you remember"		"Here's a clue. One word was a..."
			Not cued	Cued	
(1)					
Penny	Plate				
Apple	Table				
(2)					

Item	Category	Interference task	Not cued	Cued
Penny	Money	Count 1–26	2	1
Plate	Dish	Recite the alphabet A to Z	2	1
Apple	Fruit	Now pair the number with the letter as 1-a, 2-b, 3-c...	2	1
Table	Furniture	No more than 2 errors in 60 s is normal	2	1

Adapted from Buschke H, Kuslansky G, Katz M, et al. Screening for dementia with the memory impairment screen. Neurology 1999;52:231–8.

Box 4
Screen for executive dysfunction

Oral Trail Making Test part B requires the patient to count from 1 to 25 and then recite the 26 letters of the alphabet. Persons requiring greater than 60 seconds or committing 1 or more errors on either task do not have sufficient concentration to reliably complete the next step. For testing, the subject is asked to pair numbers with letters in sequence; for example, 1-A, 2-B, 3-C, and so forth, until the 13-M is reached. More than 2 errors in 13 pairings indicate impairment.

Data from Kennedy GJ, Smyth CA. Screening older adults for executive dysfunction: an essential refinement in the assessment of cognitive impairment. Am J Nurs 2008;108:62–71.

---

include measures of language, perceptual motor function, and executive function. However, because impairments in memory and executive function are thought to be among the earliest signs of dementia, screening focused on these 2 domains may be preferable. The International Association of Gerontology and Geriatrics and its Global Aging Research Network found that a combination of patient-based and informant-based screens is appropriate to detect early cognitive impairment, which may be treatable.[38] However, subsequent reviews found insufficient evidence to support or reject the use of the Mini-Cog,[39] MoCA,[40] and the collateral Informant Questionnaire on Cognitive Decline in the Elderly (IQCODE).[41]

The Memory Impairment Screen (MIS) has also been recommended.[42] It is a 4-item delayed free-recall and cued-recall test in which words are displayed to the patient who reads them aloud and is then given a category cue to facilitate recall.[43] A nonsemantic interference is then interposed before the patient is asked to recall the words (**Boxes 2** and **3, Table 5**). The MIS has been modified and validated for telephone administration (MIS-T) making it convenient for screening at the bedside or to visually impaired persons.[44] At a score of 4 or less, the MIS-T achieves a sensitivity of 78% and specificity of 93%. The MIS has also been transformed for administration with pictures (PMIS), for use with populations of low literacy.[45] It can be displayed on the desktop or handheld computer screen. It has distinguished cognitively unimpaired older adults from those with dementia regardless of differences in education, sex, age, or depression. The MIS is copyrighted by the Albert Einstein College of Medicine, which allows free use in clinical practice but requires permission for research of commercial entities.

For a nonsemantic interference task, the Oral Trail Making Test Part B (**Box 4**), which is available as an online demonstration,[46] is an established measure of executive function and validated for telephone administration. However, as with other tests of executive function, it is affected by educational level.[47] The interference task used in the PMIS validation study is counting from 1 to 20 and 20 to 1.[48] When combined, tests of memory and executive function distinguish older community residents with mild cognitive impairment from the unimpaired and are superior to the MMSE in predicting who would convert from mild impairment to dementia.[49] Executive dysfunction, as screened by the Oral Trail Making Test Part B, is also associated with hospital readmission and threatened independent living.[50]

SUMMARY

The PHQ-2, GAD-2, MIS, with the Oral Trail Making Test Part B are brief and reliable screening instruments for the most common mental illnesses of late life. Avoidable disability, family burden, and costs that result from mental and physical comorbidity make screening for common mental disorders compelling.

REFERENCES

1. O'Connor EA, Whitlock EP, Gaynes B, et al. Screening for depression in adults and older adults in primary care: an updated systematic review [Internet]. Evidence Syntheses, no. 75. Rockville (MD): Agency for Healthcare Research and Quality (US); 2009. Available at: http://www. ncbi.nlm.nih.gov/books/NBK36406/ #ch1.s7. Accessed May 2, 2017.
2. Siu AL, and the US Preventive Services Task Force (USPSTF). Screening for depression in adults US Preventive Services Task Force recommendation statement. JAMA 2016;315:380–7.
3. Kocher R, Chigurupati A. The coming battle over shared savings – primary care physicians versus specialists. N Eng J Med 2016;375:104–6.
4. Kennedy GJ. Behavioral interventions for patients with major depression and severe COPD. Am J Geriatr Psychiatry 2016;11:975–6.
5. Szanton SL, Gitlin LN. Meeting the health care financing imperative through focusing on function. The CAPABLE studies. Public Policy Aging Rep 2016;26: 106–10.
6. Annual Wellness Visit: https://www.cms.gov/Outreach-and-Education/Medicare-Learning-Network-MLN/MLNProducts/downloads/AWV_chart_ICN905706.pdf. Accessed March 6, 2017.
7. Cognitive Assessment Billing Code. Available at: http://act.alz.org/site/DocServer/ G0505_Explanatory_Guide_for_Clinicians.pdf?docID=52584. Accessed March 6, 2017.
8. Gallo JJ, Hwang S, Joo JH, et al. Multimorbidity, depression, and mortality in primary care: randomized clinical trial of an evidence-based depression care management program on mortality risk. J Gen Intern Med 2016;4:380–6.
9. Brouwers C, Christensen SB, Damen NL, et al. Antidepressant use and risk for mortality in 121,252 heart failure patients with or without a diagnosis of clinical depression. Int J Cardiol 2015;203:867–73.
10. Freedland KE, Carney RM, Rich MW, et al. Cognitive behavior therapy for depression and self-care in heart failure patients: a randomized clinical trial. JAMA Intern Med 2015;175:1773–82.
11. Beck AT, Ward CH, Mendelson M, et al. An inventory for measuring depression. Arch Gen Psychiatry 1961;4:561–71.
12. Schwab JJ, Bialow MR, Clemmons RS, et al. Hamilton rating scale for depression with medical in-patients. Br J Psychiatry 1967;113:83–8.
13. Yesavage JA, Brink TL, Rose TL, et al. Development and validation of a geriatric depression screening scale: a preliminary report. J Psychiatr Res 1982–1983;17: 37–49.
14. Doraiswamy PM, Bernstein IH, Rush AJ, et al. Diagnostic utility of the quick inventory of depressive symptomatology (QIDS-C16 and QIDS-SR16) in the elderly. Acta Psychiatr Scand 2010;122:226–34.
15. Kroenke K, Spitzer RL, Williams JB. The PHQ-9: validity of a brief depression severity measure. J Gen Intern Med 2001;16:606–13.
16. American Psychiatric Association. Desk reference to the diagnostic criteria from DSM-5. Arlington (VA): American Psychiatric Association; 2013.
17. Mitchell AJ, Yadegarfar M, Gill J, et al. Case finding and screening clinical utility of the Patient Health Questionnaire (PHQ-9 and PHQ-2) for depression in primary care: a diagnostic meta-analysis of 40 studies. BJPsych Open 2016;9:127–38.
18. Sample health risk assessment. Available at: http://www.cdc.gov/policy/hst/hra/ FrameworkForHRA.pdf. Accessed March 6, 2017.

19. Fine TH, Contractor AA, Tamburrino M, et al. Validation of the telephone-administered PHQ-9 against the in-person administered SCID-I major depression module. J Affect Disord 2013;150:1001–7.
20. Farzanfar R, Hereen T, Fava J, et al. Psychometric properties of an automated telephone-based PHQ-9. Telemed J E Health 2014;20:115–21.
21. Allen K, Cull A, Sharpe M. Diagnosing major depression in medical outpatients: acceptability of telephone interviews. J Psychosom Res 2003;55:385–7.
22. Pickett YR, Kennedy GJ, Freeman K, et al. The effect of telephone-facilitated depression care on older, medically Ill patients. J Behav Health Serv Res 2014; 41:90–6.
23. Löwe B, Schenkel IC, Carney-Doebbeling C, et al. Responsiveness of the PHQ-9 to Psychopharmacological depression treatment. Psychosomatics 2006;47:62–7.
24. Blay SL, Marinho V. Anxiety disorders in old age. Curr Opin Psychiatry 2012;25: 462–7.
25. Schuurmans J, van Balkom A. Late-life anxiety disorders. Curr Psychiatry Rep 2011;13:2267–73.
26. Cimarolli VR, Casten RV, Rovner BW, et al. Anxiety and depression in patients with advanced macular degeneration: current perspectives. Clin Ophthalmol 2016;10: 55–63.
27. Bryant C, Jackson H, Ames D. Depression and anxiety in medically unwell older adults: prevalence and short-term course. Int Psychogeriatr 2009;21:754–63.
28. Lenze EJ, Wetherell JL. A lifespan view of anxiety disorders. Dialogues Clin Neurosci 2011;13:381–99.
29. Spitzer RL, Kroenke K, Williams JB, et al. A brief measure for assessing Generalized Anxiety Disorder: the GAD-7. Arch Intern Med 2006;166:1092–7.
30. Vasiliadis HM, Chudzinski V, Gontijo-Guerra S, et al. Screening instruments for a population of older adults: the 10-item Kessler Psychological Distress Scale (K10) and the 7-item Generalized Anxiety Disorder Scale (GAD-7). Psychiatry Res 2015;228:89–94.
31. Wild B, Eckl A, Herzog W, et al. Assessing generalized anxiety disorder in elderly people using the GAD-7 and GAD-2 scales: results of a validation study. Am J Geriatr Psychiatry 2014;22:1029–38.
32. De J, Wand AP. Delirium screening: a systematic review of delirium screening tools in hospitalized patients. Gerontologist 2015;55:1079–99.
33. Moyer VA, On behalf of the U.S. Preventive Services Task Force. Screening for cognitive impairment in older adults: U.S. Preventive Services Task Force recommendation statement. Ann Intern Med 2014;160:791–7.
34. Tariq SH, Tumosa N, Chibnall JT, et al. Comparison of the Saint Louis University mental status examination and the mini-mental state examination for detecting dementia and mild neurocognitive disorder–a pilot study. Am J Geriatr Psychiatry 2006;14:900–10.
35. Nasreddine ZS, Phillips NA, Bédirian V, et al. The Montreal Cognitive Assessment, MoCA: a brief screening tool for mild cognitive impairment. J Am Geriatr Soc 2005;53:695–9.
36. Borson S, Scanlan J, Brush M, et al. The mini-cog: a cognitive 'vital signs' measure for dementia screening in multi-lingual elderly. Int J Geriatr Psychiatry 2000; 11:1021–7.
37. Creavin ST, Wisniewski S, Noel-Storr AH, et al. Mini-Mental State Examination (MMSE) for the detection of dementia in clinically unevaluated people aged 65 and over in community and primary care populations. Cochrane Database Syst Rev 2016;(1):CD011145.

38. Morley JE, Morris JC, Berg-Weger M, et al. Brain health: the importance of recognizing cognitive impairment: an IAGG consensus conference. J Am Med Dir Assoc 2015;16:731–9.
39. Fage BA, Chan CC, Gill SS, et al. Mini-Cog for the diagnosis of Alzheimer's disease dementia and other dementias within a community setting. Cochrane Database Syst Rev 2015;(2):CD010860.
40. Davis DH, Creavin ST, Yip JL, et al. Montreal Cognitive Assessment for the diagnosis of Alzheimer's disease and other dementias. Cochrane Database Syst Rev 2015;(10):CD010775.
41. Harrison JK, Stott DJ, McShane R, et al. Informant Questionnaire on Cognitive Decline in the Elderly (IQCODE) for the early diagnosis of dementia across a variety of healthcare settings. Cochrane Database Syst Rev 2016;(11):CD011333.
42. Holsinger T, Deveau J, Boustani M, et al. Does this patient have dementia? JAMA 2007;297:2391–404.
43. Buschke H, Kuslansky G, Katz M, et al. Screening for dementia with the memory impairment screen. Neurology 1999;52:231–8.
44. Lipton RB, Katz MJ, Kuslansky G, et al. Screening for dementia by telephone using the memory impairment screen. J Am Geriatr Soc 2003;51:1382–90.
45. Verghese J, Noone ML, Johnson B, et al. Picture-based memory impairment screen for dementia. J Am Geriatr Soc 2012;60:2116–20.
46. Kennedy GJ, Smyth CA. Screening older adults for executive dysfunction: an essential refinement in the assessment of cognitive impairment. Am J Nurs 2008;108:62–71.
47. Ruchinskas RA. Limitations of Oral Trail Making Test in a mixed sample of older individuals. Clin Neuropsychol 2003;17:137–42.
48. Nakata E, Kasai M, Kasuya M, et al. Combined memory and executive function tests can screen mild cognitive impairment and converters to dementia in a community: the Osaki-Tajiri project. Neuroepidemiology 2009;33:103–10.
49. Buslovich S, Kennedy GJ. Prevalence and potential impact of screening for subtle cognitive deficits on hospital readmissions. J Amer Geriatr Soc 2012;60:1980–1.
50. Cooney LM, Kennedy GJ, Hawkins KA, et al. Who can stay at home: assessing the capacity to choose to live in the community. Arch Intern Med 2004;164:357–60.

Cardiovascular Screening and Primary Prevention in Older Adults

Ariela R. Orkaby, MD, MPH[a,b,*], Michael W. Rich, MD[c]

KEYWORDS

- Cardiovascular disease • Prevention • Elderly • Aging • Statins • Hypertension
- Diabetes • Screening

KEY POINTS

- Older adults carry the highest burden of cardiovascular disease (CVD) and have the greatest potential to benefit from primary prevention strategies.
- Lifestyle strategies, including smoking cessation, physical activity, and healthy diet, are encouraged at all ages, functional levels, and cognitive stages.
- Robust older adults should be screened for CVD and have risk factors treated similar to younger adults, with attention to the increased risk for adverse effects.
- Older adults with limited life expectancy are unlikely to benefit from aggressive preventive strategies.
- Shared decision making is essential to ensure that the approach to screening and prevention is well-aligned with each patient's goals and preferences.

Although prevention of disease is a fundamental principle underlying modern medicine, evidence on appropriate preventive screening and treatment is limited for older adults. Consider the following patients scheduled to see their primary care physicians for their annual visits:

Mr K is a widowed 82-year-old living independently in the community with hypertension, hyperlipidemia, diabetes, and arthritis. He takes aspirin 81 mg, hydrochlorothiazide 25 mg, and simvastatin 40 mg daily, with ibuprofen 400 mg as needed for pain. Since his wife died a year ago he increasingly eats frozen dinners or take out, although his daughter encourages him to "eat healthy." He is a retired construction worker and

Disclosure Statement: Dr A.R. Orkaby has no relevant financial disclosures. Dr M.W. Rich has no relevant financial disclosures.
[a] Preventive Cardiology, Geriatric Research, Education, and Clinical Center (GRECC), VA Boston Healthcare System, 150 South Huntington Street, Boston, MA 02130, USA; [b] Medicine, Division of Aging, Brigham and Women's Hospital, Harvard Medical School, 1620 Tremont Street, Boston, MA 02120, USA; [c] Washington University School of Medicine, 660 Euclid Avenue, Campus Box 8086, St Louis, MO 63110, USA
* Corresponding author. 150 South Huntington Street, Boston, MA 02130.
E-mail address: Ariela.Orkaby@mail.harvard.edu

Clin Geriatr Med 34 (2018) 81–93
https://doi.org/10.1016/j.cger.2017.08.003
0749-0690/18/Published by Elsevier Inc.

geriatric.theclinics.com

spends his days doing small projects in his community. He walks his dog daily for 15 minutes and has had no falls. He smokes half a pack of cigarettes daily (down from 2 packs a day) and drinks 3 beers on the weekend. Physical examination reveals a regular heart rate of 72, blood pressure (BP) 151/78 mm Hg sitting and 153/80 mm Hg standing, and a normal gait while walking to the examination room. Laboratory data include a hemoglobin A1c (HbA1c) level of 7.2% and low-density lipoprotein (LDL)-cholesterol of 110 mg/dL.

Mr L is an 83-year-old with hypertension, hyperlipidemia, diabetes, and arthritis who recently moved to a memory unit because of gradually worsening dementia. Daily medications are aspirin 81 mg, donepezil 5 mg, lisinopril 10 mg, metformin 1000 mg, simvastatin 40 mg, and a multivitamin, with ibuprofen 400 mg as needed for pain. He has had increasing difficulty dressing himself, and requires cueing for bathing (Fast stage 6b, moderately severe dementia). He is a retired plumber and smoked half a pack of cigarettes daily until 2 years ago. He does not drink alcohol and until admission to the memory unit enjoyed going for long walks in the evenings. He has fallen once in the past month and 3 times in the past year, without significant injury. His heart rate is 64 and regular, BP 123/68 mm Hg sitting and 118/64 mm Hg standing. His gait is slow and cautious. The HbA1c is 6.2% and LDL-cholesterol is 110 mg/dL.

These 2 individuals have similar cardiovascular risk profiles, but Mr K is a robust older adult whereas Mr L has substantive functional and cognitive impairments. Considering their age alone, each has a life expectancy of approximately 7 years (US census data). Mr K, however, is independent without a life-limiting chronic disease and has an excellent prospect of living at least 7 more years, whereas Mr L has moderately severe dementia now requiring nursing home–level care with a life expectancy of only approximately 2 years.[1]

In this article, we review screening tests and prevention strategies that may be considered for primary prevention of cardiovascular disease (CVD) in older adults, with a focus on those ≥75 years of age, accounting for age, functional status, and medical conditions.

EPIDEMIOLOGY OF CARDIOVASCULAR DISEASE AND AGING

With improvements in medicine and technology, life expectancy has increased substantially over the past century. The age group 65 to 74 years is experiencing rapid growth, while the proportional rate of rise is greatest in the subgroup older than 85.[2] The incidence and prevalence of most CVDs, including ischemic heart disease, heart failure, valve disease, rhythm disorders, and stroke, rise progressively with age, and CVD remains the leading cause of death in those older than 75 years.[3] Although globally the rate of acute myocardial infarctions has decreased since 1990, the prevalence of ischemic heart disease has increased as the population has aged.[4] In the United States, according to National Health and Nutrition Examination Survey (NHANES) data from 2011 to 2014, 92.1 million adults have at least 1 type of CVD, equivalent to 1 in 3 Americans.[3] In men and women older than 80 years, the prevalence of CVD approaches 85%.[3] The patients described in the vignettes are fairly typical of those seen in daily practice: surviving into advanced age with multiple comorbidities and taking multiple medications. However, although the oldest patients carry most of the CVD burden, such patients have been markedly underrepresented in most CVD prevention trials that provide the principal evidence for CVD prevention guidelines.[5]

Some challenges to implementing CVD prevention strategies for older adults include difficulty in estimating life expectancy and clinicians' discomfort with prognostication. However, because older patients are at greater risk than younger individuals, not only for CVD events but also for adverse outcomes from such events (eg, mortality after myocardial infarction increases exponentially with age), the potential benefits of preventive therapies are also greater. Therefore, it is a disservice not to consider relevant screening and prevention strategies for CVD in older adults.

SCREENING FOR CARDIOVASCULAR DISEASE

Screening must begin with a detailed history focused on symptoms. Men and women may experience different symptoms and older adults may not report typical cardiovascular (CV) symptoms, or may not recall symptoms due to cognitive impairment.[6] It is therefore important to perform a detailed review of systems that asks not only about chest discomfort, dyspnea, palpitations, and claudication, but also assesses changes in activity level and inquires about falls or near falls, as these events may be manifestations of angina, heart failure, arrhythmias, or valve disease. Corroboration from caregivers and family members is also important, especially in patients with cognitive impairment.

In addition to assessing vital signs and body habitus, the physical examination should include palpation of pulses. The US Preventive Services Task Force (USPSTF) found no evidence to suggest that auscultation for carotid bruits is beneficial and does not recommend screening for carotid artery stenosis in asymptomatic individuals.[7] Routine screening for CVD with a resting or exercise electrocardiogram in asymptomatic patients is also not recommended.[8,9]

In men who have smoked or have had a first-degree relative with an abdominal aortic aneurysm (AAA), current USPSTF guidelines recommend a 1-time screen with ultrasound for those ages 65 to 75.[10] For older men who have never been screened, and for all women, screening should be "individualized." For a healthy 80-year-old with a 10-year life expectancy who has never been screened, offering a 1-time screen to former smokers is reasonable.

ESTIMATING RISK OF CARDIOVASCULAR DISEASE

Current risk assessment tools, such as the Framingham risk score and 2013 Atherosclerotic CVD (ASCVD) risk calculator, are not validated in individuals older than 80 years. In fact, using the 2013 ASCVD risk calculator, almost all men older than 70 and women older than 75 with no risk factors other than age are at moderate risk for CVD and are potential candidates for statin therapy.[11] None of the existing CVD risk calculators incorporate issues of aging, such as multimorbidity, cognitive impairment, functional limitations, or frailty. Furthermore, life expectancy is not accounted for in any of the existing CVD risk scores. As chronologic age may be less useful in discriminating risk in the aging population, there is growing interest in the role of markers of biological aging, such as frailty and function, in identifying individuals at heightened risk for CVD. For example, slow walking speed is a marker of frailty and vulnerability that has been associated with an increased risk for CVD.[12]

PRIMARY PREVENTION OF CARDIOVASCULAR DISEASE

Risk factors for vascular disease are typically considered in 2 categories: nonmodifiable and modifiable. Currently, age, sex, genetics, and family history are nonmodifiable risk factors. Age is the strongest risk factor for CVD, and the sex-related differences in risk seen among younger individuals become less pronounced with age.[6]

MODIFIABLE RISK FACTORS

A review of current American College of Cardiology and American Heart Association (ACC/AHA) guidelines revealed a paucity of evidence across all CVD risk factors to guide appropriate preventive strategies in older adults.[13] Of particular concern is the lack of attention to issues that are important to patients, such as maintaining independence, quality of life, and physical function.[13] Furthermore, by design, guidelines focus on specific conditions, such as heart failure or atrial fibrillation, and do not generally consider the complexities of multimorbidity and how an individual patient may be expected to follow numerous and often conflicting recommendations.

LIFESTYLE
Smoking

Although smoking rates continue to decrease, smoking remains the leading modifiable risk factor for CVD worldwide. Data suggest that smoking cessation is beneficial at all ages.[14] Strong evidence supports recommendations that all patients should be asked about tobacco habits, that smokers should be advised to quit, and smoking cessation support should be offered.[15,16] Strategies include motivational interviewing, behavioral interventions, and support groups. Pharmacotherapy with nicotine replacement and other medications may be necessary to support smoking cessation efforts and can be used safely in older patients.

Exercise

Physical activity is one of the most important preventive strategies for healthy aging and prevention of CVD.[3] All older adults benefit from increasing physical activity,[17] including those with dementia. The Lifestyle Interventions and Independence for Elders (LIFE) study compared a structured exercise regimen with health education in 818 community-dwelling older adults aged 70 to 89 years and demonstrated an 18% reduction in major mobility disability (hazard ratio [HR] 0.82, 95% confidence interval [CI] 0.69–0.98, $P = .03$).[18] Cross-sectional analysis found that physical inactivity at baseline in LIFE study participants was associated with an increased risk of CV events. However, after the trial was completed, no statistically significant difference was found in the secondary outcome of CV events (composite of myocardial infarction [MI], stroke, or CV death) (HR 1.05, 95% CI 0.67–1.66, $P = .83$).[19] The trialists conjectured that this may have been due to the choice of comparison group, which was a support group that received healthy lifestyle education. It is also possible that healthy exercise habits need to begin earlier in life, although observational studies have shown that initiating an exercise program, even at a very low level, is associated with improved outcomes, including among very elderly individuals.[20]

The ideal exercise plan for older patients must be feasible and realistic, and should include 5 components[21]:

1. Aerobic activity at least 5 days a week, ideally for 30-minute intervals. However even 10-minute intervals are beneficial, and any activity is better than no activity![20]
2. Resistance training at least 3 times a week.
3. Stretching at least 3 times a week.
4. Balance training at least 3 times a week. This can include activities such as Tai Chi or simple chair stands done in the home.
5. Encouragement of daily physical activity and avoidance of excessive sedentary behavior, such as watching television for prolonged periods.

Diet

Poor dietary habits lead to glucose intolerance, diabetes, obesity, elevated BP, and subsequent rise in CV events.[3] General improvements in healthy diet have been noted across the United States in the past decade, in large part due to a reduction in sugar-sweetened beverage intake and increase in whole grains.[3] The PREDIMED trial, undertaken in 7447 adults in Spain aged 50 to 80 years, demonstrated a protective effect of the Mediterranean diet supplemented with olive oil or nuts. Compared with a low-fat diet, the intervention diets reduced major CV events by 30% (HR 0.70, 95% CI 0.54–0.92).[22] A balanced diet that includes fruits, vegetables, whole grains, nuts, lean proteins, and healthy fats (polyunsaturated fatty acids) is recommended. In older individuals, malnutrition due to cognitive impairment, limited mobility and access to food, lack of social support, poor dentition, and frailty may make it difficult to achieve an ideal diet; nonetheless, a healthy diet should be encouraged.

RISK FACTORS
Hypertension

The prevalence of hypertension rises with age, with estimates that more than 75% of those $\geq$80 years have hypertension.[3] The most common form of hypertension in older adults is isolated systolic hypertension. The 2014 Eighth Joint National Committee (JNC8) guidelines on hypertension management were based primarily on data from randomized controlled trials and concluded that limited data were available to define optimal BP goals for older adults.[23] The result was a recommended BP goal of less than 150/90 mm Hg for those older than 60 years, and less than 140/90 mm Hg in those with diabetes.

On the other hand, meta-analysis of individual patient-level data from 61 studies, including 1 million adults without CVD, has demonstrated a consistent decrease in mortality and CV events with lower BPs, even as low as 115 mm Hg, at all ages.[24] The Hypertension in the Very Elderly Trial (HYVET) randomized 3845 participants older than 80 years with systolic BP (SBP) 160 to 199 mm Hg to indapamide or placebo with a goal BP <150/90 mm Hg.[25] The trial was stopped early after demonstrating a significant reduction in stroke and mortality.

The recently completed Systolic Blood Pressure Intervention Trial (SPRINT) adds to the evidence for older adults and calls the JNC8 guideline into question.[26] SPRINT randomized 9361 participants older than 50 years with baseline SBP 130 to 180 mm Hg to a goal SBP less than 140 mm Hg versus <120 mm Hg. The main trial results demonstrated a significant 25% reduction in major CV events (HR 0.75, CI 0.64–0.89) and 27% reduction in mortality (HR 0.73, CI 0.60–0.90). In a prespecified subgroup of participants older than 75 years (n = 2636) the results were even more striking, with a 34% reduction in CVD events (HR 0.66, CI 0.51–0.85) and 33% reduction in mortality (HR 0.67, CI 0.49–0.91).[27] The greater benefit in older patients likely reflects the higher burden of CVD in this population.

Importantly, SPRINT is the first hypertension trial to consider the role of frailty, measured using both gait speed and a cumulative deficit model.[28] Overall, 30% of trial participants were identified as frail using either measure. Benefits of BP reduction were seen regardless of frailty status or walking speed. Reanalysis of HYVET considering frailty also demonstrated consistent benefit of lowering BP even in frail individuals.[29]

Although these results from SPRINT are important and should be incorporated into hypertension management guidelines for older adults, there are important caveats to consider before translation into routine practice. Participants in SPRINT were generally healthier than those seen in the community. To be included in the trial, participants had to have a life expectancy of more than 3 years and not have diabetes (due to the parallel ACCORD [Action to Control Cardiovascular Disease in Diabetes] trial[30]), heart failure, dementia, nursing home residence, or "poor compliance." Although frailty rates were similar to those reported in the community, the mortality rate in the frail cohort was lower than expected.[31] Further, BP measurement in a clinical trial (done in a quiet room after the participant has been sitting for 5 minutes) may not mirror typical clinic BPs. Finally, rates of serious adverse events, including electrolyte abnormalities, syncope, hypotension, and acute kidney injury in the intensive treatment group were significantly higher than in the usual care group, although these differences did not achieve statistical significance in the subgroup of those older than 75 years, possibly due to smaller sample size and lack of power.

Since 2012, the American Diabetes Association (ADA) in conjunction with the American Geriatrics Society has advocated incorporating functional status and life expectancy into its recommendations. In individuals with diabetes, the ADA suggests for those who are relatively healthy or with only a few medical conditions, a BP goal of lower than 140/90 mm Hg is appropriate, regardless of age.[32] For those with functional limitation or limited life expectancy, a less-aggressive goal of lower than 150/90 mm Hg is appropriate. Canadian guidelines suggest a goal of lower than 160/90 mm Hg may be most appropriate for frail individuals.

In summary, all older adults should be screened for hypertension, with BP measured in both the sitting and standing positions to evaluate for orthostatic hypotension and associated symptoms. Treatment should be considered in those with BP >150/90 mm Hg, regardless of frailty or functional status. For those with frailty, functional limitation, or frequent falls, care must be taken to avoid orthostasis, perhaps treating to standing BP or using small doses of several medications rather than a single high-dose medication. Careful uptitration of medication with attention to side effects and drug-drug interactions is essential.

Hypercholesterolemia

Elevated cholesterol is an established risk factor for CVD in young and middle-age populations. With aging, the role of elevated cholesterol is less clear. Low cholesterol may reflect underlying malnutrition, malignancy, or frailty, whereas elevated cholesterol has been associated with longevity.[33]

The 2013 ACC/AHA guideline[11] notes that there are limited data on treatment of cholesterol for the primary prevention of CVD in individuals older than 75 years. This is a direct result of the lack of inclusion of older individuals in cardiovascular trials. In one meta-analysis of 170,000 participants in statin trials, fewer than 2% were older than 75 years.[34] The Prospective Study of Pravastatin in the Elderly at Risk (PROSPER) randomized 5804 participants aged 70 to 82 years with or without a history of CVD to pravastatin or placebo.[35] After a mean follow-up of 3 years, a significant 15% reduction in major CVD events was seen (HR 0.85, 95% CI 0.74–0.97), although the benefit appeared to be limited to those with prior CVD ($P = .19$ for interaction). Exploratory analysis of the Justification for the Use of Statins in Primary Prevention (JUPITER) trial focused on 5695 individuals older than 70 years randomized to rosuvastatin versus placebo and found a significant reduction in all-cause mortality and major CVD events (HR 0.61, 95% CI 0.46–0.82).[36] Neither trial enrolled many participants older than 80 years. Additionally, the absolute benefit in JUPITER was low, with an absolute risk reduction (ARR) of 0.77% for the primary endpoint (number needed to treat [NNT] 130) and an ARR of 0.41% for all-cause mortality (NNT 244).

Recently published secondary analysis of the 2867 participants older than 65 years randomized to pravastatin versus placebo in the Antihypertensive and Lipid-Lowering Treatment to Prevent Heart Attack Trial–Lipid-Lowering Trial (ALLHAT-LLT) adds to the uncertainty about the role of statins for primary prevention in older adults. No benefit was found for CVD reduction or all-cause mortality. Focusing on the 726 individuals older than 75 years followed for 6 years, there was no significant difference in MI or fatal MI (HR 0.70, 95% CI 0.43–1.13, $P = .14$), with a nonsignificant increased risk of mortality in those taking pravastatin (HR 1.34, 95% CI 0.98–1.84, $P = .097$). A major caveat of this analysis was the high rate of crossover between the intervention and control group and the relatively low number of participants older than 75 years that precluded drawing meaningful conclusions.[37]

The ACC/AHA guideline recommends that physicians and patients engage in shared decision making when deciding on whether statin therapy is appropriate. As noted previously, with current risk calculators all individuals older than 80 years are at least moderate risk due to age alone. However, chronologic age is often not reflective of biological age in older adults and may lead to underestimation or overestimation of life expectancy. Measures such as self-paced gait speed over a short distance (4–10 m) may provide additional insight into life expectancy and help guide decision-making.[12]

In weighing risks and benefits of statins, important issues to consider are comorbid conditions, drug-drug interactions, and side effects. Data are limited on the risks of statins in those older than 75 years, but there may be an increased risk of functional and cognitive decline.[38] Time to benefit for statins for primary prevention is estimated at 2 to 5 years.[39] Therefore, an individual with a life-limiting illness is unlikely to benefit from a statin for primary prevention and may in fact benefit from deprescribing.[40]

Given the limited evidence for statins for primary prevention in those older than 80 years, it is reasonable to offer a statin to those with good functional status and an estimated life expectancy of at least 2 years. It is prudent to begin with a low dose of a low-potency statin with slow uptitration while carefully monitoring for symptoms of myalgia and fatigue.

Diabetes Mellitus

Diabetes is a major risk factor for CVD and has been considered a CVD "risk equivalent." The prevalence of diabetes is 20% in those older than 65 years and is expected to rise due to increasing rates of obesity.[32] Although recent studies of novel antidiabetic agents, such as canagliflozin, a sodium-glucose cotransporter 2 inhibitor, have shown beneficial effects on reducing CVD outcomes,[41] very few individuals older than 75 were included, and there is a lack of evidence demonstrating that diabetes control at any level reduces CVD risk in older adults.[42]

Management goals for diabetes in older patients updated by the ADA now incorporate issues of function, life expectancy, and anticipated benefit from treatment.[32] The guidelines emphasize overall health and functional status in making recommendations for hemoglobin A1c (Hb A1c) goals. For those who are relatively healthy with few medical conditions that are well controlled, a goal Hb A1c <7.5% is reasonable. For individuals with multiple chronic conditions, or with either mild cognitive impairment or difficulty with more than 2 activities of daily living, an Hb A1c goal less than 8.0% is recommended. In those with limited life expectancy, end-stage illness, or moderate to severe cognitive impairment or functional limitation, an Hb A1c goal of less than 8.5% should be considered. The guidelines point out that although avoidance of hypoglycemia is paramount, hyperglycemia also should be avoided, although without specific guidance as to what is acceptable beyond Hb A1c goals. Overall, emphasis is on individualizing the diabetes care plan.

Frailty

Frailty is increasingly recognized as both a risk factor for CVD and as an outcome of CVD events.[43] Whether frailty is a modifiable risk factor for CVD remains unknown. However, intriguing data suggest that individuals who are at risk of frailty are also at risk for CVD, implying a shared pathogenesis.[44] Measurement of gait speed is a simple tool to screen for frailty and should be considered as part of the standard physical examination in all older adults. Pooled data from 9 cohort studies involving 34,485 patients demonstrated a strong association between gait speed and mortality, and a 0.1 m/s increment in gait speed was associated with a 10% reduction in 1-year mortality.[45]

Gait speed integrates multiple organ systems, so it is perhaps not surprising that faster gait is associated with lower mortality. CVD prevention strategies, particularly exercise, may help improve gait speed and mobility, as demonstrated by the LIFE trial. However, although the presence of frailty identifies a population of older adults at increased risk for CVD, whether aggressive preventive interventions can lead to improved outcomes in these individuals remains to be established.

PHARMACOLOGIC INTERVENTIONS

Aspirin

The role of antiplatelet therapy for primary prevention in older adults remains uncertain. Meta-analytic data suggest a modest reduction in the risk of nonfatal MI without significant effects on nonfatal stroke or CV death.[46] A randomized trial of low-dose aspirin for the primary prevention of CVD in adults 60 to 85 years undertaken in Japan failed to show a reduction in CV events.[47] Important caveats in interpreting this trial are that event rates were lower than expected, crossover rates were high, rates of hemorrhagic stroke were greater than reported in Western studies, and the trial may have been underpowered to detect a beneficial effect of aspirin.[48]

The 2016 USPSTF report on aspirin found that for those ≥70 years, evidence was inconclusive but pointed toward harm, principally because the risk of bleeding increases with age.[49] Due to the lack of evidence of benefit and significant concern for harm, current guidelines on appropriate medication use in older adults both from Europe and the American Geriatrics Society's Beers Criteria do not recommend aspirin for primary prevention in those older than 80 years, even in patients with diabetes.[50,51] It is anticipated that the ongoing Aspirin in Reducing Events in Elderly (ASPREE) trial will shed further light on this important issue.[52]

Angiotensin-Converting Enzyme Inhibitors/Angiotensin II Receptor Blockers

There is growing interest in the role of renin-angiotensin-aldosterone system blockers for primary prevention of CVD. Angiotensin-converting enzyme inhibitors (ACEIs) and angiotensin II receptor blockers (ARBs) are established therapies for secondary prevention of CVD, due to their effects in reducing neuro-hormonal activation, oxidative stress, platelet activation, and vascular remodeling.[53] For primary prevention, the Heart Outcomes Prevention Evaluation, which randomized 9297 patients ≥55 years of age to ramipril or placebo, found that the benefits of ramipril in reducing CVD events were similar among patients with or without preexisting CVD.[54] In part for this reason, ACEIs are considered first-line therapy for hypertension management in patients with systolic heart failure, diabetes, or chronic kidney disease, including older adults.[23,32] Although ARBs are frequently used as an alternative to ACEIs, it is unclear that they are as safe and effective as ACEIs in older adults.[55] Interestingly, there is a growing body of evidence to suggest that ACEIs may help prevent frailty by slowing age-related muscle loss and improving exercise capacity.[56] Further work is needed to understand the role of ACEIs and ARBs in primary prevention of CVD in older adults.

RECOMMENDATIONS

Mr K is a relatively healthy 82-year-old with an estimated life expectancy longer than 5 years who is likely to benefit from primary CVD prevention strategies. He should be counseled to quit smoking and offered nicotine replacement treatment if necessary. If he has not had a 1-time screen for AAA, this should be discussed. He should be encouraged to increase his physical activity, perhaps by increasing the duration of

Table 1
Considerations for screening and treatment for the primary prevention of cardiovascular disease for adults older than 75 years

	Community Dwelling, Functioning Near Independent, Mild Frailty, Life Expectancy >3–5 y	Frail, Advanced Dementia, Institutionalized, or Limited Life Expectancy <2 y
Screening		
History and physical	Always	Always
Routine electrocardiogram or stress testing	Not recommended	Not recommended
Carotid artery stenosis	Not recommended	Not recommended
Abdominal aortic aneurysm	Ever smoker: consider screening	Not recommended
Cardiovascular disease risk prediction tool	Not validated in those >80 y	
Prevention strategies		
Smoking cessation	Always	Always
Physical activity	Always (1) Aerobic activity, (2) stretching, (3) resistance, (4) balance training	Always (1) Aerobic activity, (2) stretching, (3) resistance, (4) balance training
Dietary review	Always	Always
Hypertension	Screen: Always Treat to goal <150/90, consider <140/90 with attention to adverse effects	Screen: Always If life expectancy >6 mo, consider treating to goal <150/90
Hypercholesterolemia	Screen: Not recommended Treatment: Offer low-dose, low-intensity statin (eg, pravastatin 10 mg), monitor for adverse reactions	Screen: Not recommended Treatment: Not recommended, consider deprescribing if taking a statin
Diabetes	Screen: Annually Treat to goal A1c <7.5%–8.0%	Screen: Annually Treat to goal A1c <8.0%–8.5%
Frailty	Always	Always
Pharmacologic interventions		
Aspirin	Not recommended	Not recommended
Angiotensin-converting enzyme inhibitors	First line for hypertension management in those with systolic heart failure, diabetes, or chronic kidney disease	

his daily walk to 20 to 30 minutes and adding balance and resistance exercises. He may benefit from consultation with a nutritionist to improve his food choices and lower his salt intake. Review of his medications reveals a nonsteroidal anti-inflammatory drug that may be contributing to his hypertension as well as his overall CVD risk.[57] If his arthritic pain is well controlled, he could consider stopping this medication or trying acetaminophen as an alternative. Hydrochlorothiazide may increase the risk of electrolyte abnormalities and falls; a low-dose ACEI would be more appropriate, especially given his history of diabetes. Because his diabetes is well controlled for his age, he does not need additional therapy beyond diet and exercise.

Mr L has moderately severe dementia with limited life expectancy of less than 2 years and slow gait, suggesting physical frailty. He is unlikely to live long enough to benefit from a statin or aspirin and consideration should be given to stopping both. His Hb A1c is well below the recommended target for his age and health status; hence, metformin should be stopped. His BP is also well below the goal of less than 150/90 given his functional status, and particularly considering his falls he would likely benefit from looser BP control. He should be encouraged to remain physically active, but evaluation for an assistive device, such as a cane or walker, should be considered to reduce the risk of falls. His family should be engaged in the decision-making process, as he is unlikely to be able to advocate for himself because of his dementia.

SUMMARY

Screening for CVD and application of primary prevention strategies in the very old should incorporate life expectancy, time to benefit, and individual goals. Additional factors to consider include physical and cognitive function, comorbidity and medication burden, and frailty. A shared decision-making process is essential to ensure that the approach to screening and prevention is well-aligned with each patient's goals and preferences. **Table 1** provides a summary of recommendations for screening and prevention strategies that may serve as a starting point for such discussions.

REFERENCES

1. Wolfson C, Wolfson DB, Asgharian M, et al. A reevaluation of the duration of survival after the onset of dementia. N Engl J Med 2001;344(15):1111–6.
2. Available at: http://www.pgpf.org/chart-archive/0045_elderly-population-trends. Accessed April 24, 2017.
3. Benjamin EJ, Blaha MJ, Chiuve SE, et al. Heart disease and stroke statistics-2017 update: a report from the American Heart Association. Circulation 2017;135(10): e146–603.
4. Moran AE, Forouzanfar MH, Roth GA, et al. The global burden of ischemic heart disease in 1990 and 2010: the Global Burden of Disease 2010 study. Circulation 2014;129(14):1493–501.
5. Alexander KP, Newby LK, Cannon CP, et al. Acute coronary care in the elderly, part I: non-ST-segment-elevation acute coronary syndromes: a scientific statement for healthcare professionals from the American Heart Association Council on Clinical Cardiology: in collaboration with the Society of Geriatric Cardiology. Circulation 2007;115(19):2549–69.
6. Peterson E, Gharacholou S. Coronary heart disease. Hazzard's geriatric medicine and gerontology. New York: The McGraw-Hill Companies, Inc; 2009. p. 909–19.
7. LeFevre ML. Screening for asymptomatic carotid artery stenosis: U.S. Preventive Services Task Force recommendation statement. Ann Intern Med 2014;161(5): 356–62.

8. Gibbons RJ, Balady GJ, Bricker JT, et al. ACC/AHA 2002 guideline update for exercise testing: summary article. A report of the American College of Cardiology/American Heart Association Task Force on Practice Guidelines (Committee to update the 1997 exercise testing guidelines). J Am Coll Cardiol 2002;40(8): 1531–40.

9. Moyer VA. Screening for coronary heart disease with electrocardiography: U.S. Preventive Services Task Force recommendation statement. Ann Intern Med 2012;157(7):512–8.

10. LeFevre ML. Screening for abdominal aortic aneurysm: U.S. Preventive Services Task Force recommendation statement. Ann Intern Med 2014;161(4):281–90.

11. Stone NJ, Robinson JG, Lichtenstein AH, et al. 2013 ACC/AHA guideline on the treatment of blood cholesterol to reduce atherosclerotic cardiovascular risk in adults: a report of the American College of Cardiology/American Heart Association Task Force on Practice Guidelines. J Am Coll Cardiol 2014;63(25 Pt B): 2889–934.

12. Afilalo J, Karunananthan S, Eisenberg MJ, et al. Role of frailty in patients with cardiovascular disease. Am J Cardiol 2009;103(11):1616–21.

13. Rich MW, Chyun DA, Skolnick AH, et al. Knowledge gaps in cardiovascular care of the older adult population: a scientific statement from the American Heart Association, American College of Cardiology, and American Geriatrics Society. Circulation 2016;133(21):2103–22.

14. Taylor DH Jr, Hasselblad V, Henley SJ, et al. Benefits of smoking cessation for longevity. Am J Public Health 2002;92(6):990–6.

15. 2008 PHS Guideline Update Panel, Liaisons, and Staff. Treating tobacco use and dependence: 2008 update U.S. Public Health Service Clinical Practice Guideline executive summary. Respir Care 2008;53(9):1217–22.

16. Siu AL. Behavioral and pharmacotherapy interventions for tobacco smoking cessation in adults, including pregnant women: U.S. Preventive Services Task Force recommendation statement. Ann Intern Med 2015;163(8):622–34.

17. Villareal DT, Chode S, Parimi N, et al. Weight loss, exercise, or both and physical function in obese older adults. N Engl J Med 2011;364(13):1218–29.

18. Pahor M, Guralnik JM, Ambrosius WT, et al. Effect of structured physical activity on prevention of major mobility disability in older adults: the LIFE study randomized clinical trial. JAMA 2014;311(23):2387–96.

19. Newman AB, Dodson JA, Church TS, et al. Cardiovascular events in a physical activity intervention compared with a successful aging intervention: the LIFE study randomized trial. JAMA Cardiol 2016;1(5):568–74.

20. Powell KE, Paluch AE, Blair SN. Physical activity for health: what kind? How much? How intense? On top of what? Annu Rev Public Health 2011;32:349–65.

21. Elsawy B, Higgins KE. Physical activity guidelines for older adults. Am Fam Physician 2010;81(1):55–9.

22. Estruch R, Ros E, Salas-Salvado J, et al. Primary prevention of cardiovascular disease with a Mediterranean diet. N Engl J Med 2013;368(14):1279–90.

23. James PA, Oparil S, Carter BL, et al. 2014 evidence-based guideline for the management of high blood pressure in adults: report from the panel members appointed to the Eighth Joint National Committee (JNC 8). JAMA 2014;311(5): 507–20.

24. Lewington S, Clarke R, Qizilbash N, et al. Age-specific relevance of usual blood pressure to vascular mortality: a meta-analysis of individual data for one million adults in 61 prospective studies. Lancet 2002;360(9349):1903–13.

25. Beckett NS, Peters R, Fletcher AE, et al. Treatment of hypertension in patients 80 years of age or older. N Engl J Med 2008;358(18):1887–98.
26. Wright JT Jr, Williamson JD, Whelton PK, et al. A randomized trial of intensive versus standard blood-pressure control. N Engl J Med 2015;373(22):2103–16.
27. Williamson JD, Supiano MA, Applegate WB, et al. Intensive vs standard blood pressure control and cardiovascular disease outcomes in adults aged >/=75 years: a randomized clinical trial. JAMA 2016;315(24):2673–82.
28. Pajewski NM, Williamson JD, Applegate WB, et al. Characterizing frailty status in the systolic blood pressure intervention trial. J Gerontol A Biol Sci Med Sci 2016; 71(5):649–55.
29. Warwick J, Falaschetti E, Rockwood K, et al. No evidence that frailty modifies the positive impact of antihypertensive treatment in very elderly people: an investigation of the impact of frailty upon treatment effect in the HYpertension in the Very Elderly Trial (HYVET) study, a double-blind, placebo-controlled study of antihypertensives in people with hypertension aged 80 and over. BMC Med 2015;13:78.
30. Cushman WC, Evans GW, Byington RP, et al. Effects of intensive blood-pressure control in type 2 diabetes mellitus. N Engl J Med 2010;362(17):1575–85.
31. Kim DH. Intensive vs standard blood pressure control for older adults. JAMA 2016;316(18):1921.
32. American Diabetes Association. 11. Older adults. Diabetes Care 2017; 40(Supplement 1):S99–104.
33. Newson RS, Felix JF, Heeringa J, et al. Association between serum cholesterol and noncardiovascular mortality in older age. J Am Geriatr Soc 2011;59(10): 1779–85.
34. Cholesterol Treatment Trialists' (CTT) Collaboration, Baigent C, Blackwell L, Emberson J, et al. Efficacy and safety of more intensive lowering of LDL cholesterol: a meta-analysis of data from 170,000 participants in 26 randomised trials. Lancet 2010;376(9753):1670–81.
35. Shepherd J, Blauw GJ, Murphy MB, et al. Pravastatin in elderly individuals at risk of vascular disease (PROSPER): a randomised controlled trial. Lancet 2002; 360(9346):1623–30.
36. Glynn RJ, Koenig W, Nordestgaard BG, et al. Rosuvastatin for primary prevention in older persons with elevated C-reactive protein and low to average low-density lipoprotein cholesterol levels: exploratory analysis of a randomized trial. Ann Intern Med 2010;152:488–96. W174.
37. Han BH, Sutin D, Williamson JD, et al. Effect of statin treatment vs usual care on primary cardiovascular prevention among older adults: the ALLHAT-LLT randomized clinical trial. JAMA Intern Med 2017;177(7):955–65.
38. Odden MC, Pletcher MJ, Coxson PG, et al. Cost-effectiveness and population impact of statins for primary prevention in adults aged 75 years or older in the United States. Ann Intern Med 2015;162(8):533–41.
39. Holmes HM, Min LC, Yee M, et al. Rationalizing prescribing for older patients with multimorbidity: considering time to benefit. Drugs Aging 2013;30(9):655–66.
40. Kutner JS, Blatchford PJ, Taylor DH Jr, et al. Safety and benefit of discontinuing statin therapy in the setting of advanced, life-limiting illness: a randomized clinical trial. JAMA Intern Med 2015;175(5):691–700.
41. Neal B, Perkovic V, Mahaffey KW, et al. Canagliflozin and cardiovascular and renal events in type 2 diabetes. N Engl J Med 2017;377(7):644–57.
42. Halter JB, Musi N, McFarland Horne F, et al. Diabetes and cardiovascular disease in older adults: current status and future directions. Diabetes 2014;63(8): 2578–89.

43. Afilalo J, Alexander KP, Mack MJ, et al. Frailty assessment in the cardiovascular care of older adults. J Am Coll Cardiol 2014;63(8):747–62.
44. Ricci NA, Pessoa GS, Ferriolli E, et al. Frailty and cardiovascular risk in community-dwelling elderly: a population-based study. Clin Interv Aging 2014; 9:1677–85.
45. Studenski S, Perera S, Patel K, et al. Gait speed and survival in older adults. JAMA 2011;305(1):50–8.
46. Baigent C, Blackwell L, Collins R, et al. Aspirin in the primary and secondary prevention of vascular disease: collaborative meta-analysis of individual participant data from randomised trials. Lancet 2009;373:1849–60.
47. Ikeda Y, Shimada K, Teramoto T, et al. Low-dose aspirin for primary prevention of cardiovascular events in Japanese patients 60 years or older with atherosclerotic risk factors: a randomized clinical trial. JAMA 2014;312(23):2510–20.
48. Gaziano JM, Greenland P. When should aspirin be used for prevention of cardiovascular events? JAMA 2014;312:2503–4.
49. Bibbins-Domingo K. Aspirin use for the primary prevention of cardiovascular disease and colorectal cancer: U.S. Preventive Services Task Force recommendation statement. Ann Intern Med 2016;164(12):836–45.
50. By the American Geriatrics Society 2015 Beers Criteria Update Expert Panel. American Geriatrics Society 2015 updated beers criteria for potentially inappropriate medication use in older adults. J Am Geriatr Soc 2015;63(11):2227–46.
51. O'Mahony D, O'Sullivan D, Byrne S, et al. STOPP/START criteria for potentially inappropriate prescribing in older people: version 2. Age Ageing 2015;44(2): 213–8.
52. ASPREE Investigator Group. Study design of ASPirin in Reducing Events in the Elderly (ASPREE): a randomized, controlled trial. Contemp Clin Trials 2013; 36(2):555–64.
53. Smith SC Jr, Benjamin EJ, Bonow RO, et al. AHA/ACCF secondary prevention and risk reduction therapy for patients with coronary and other atherosclerotic vascular disease: 2011 update: a guideline from the American Heart Association and American College of Cardiology Foundation. Circulation 2011;124(22): 2458–73.
54. Yusuf S, Sleight P, Pogue J, et al. Effects of an angiotensin-converting-enzyme inhibitor, ramipril, on cardiovascular events in high-risk patients. N Engl J Med 2000;342(3):145–53.
55. Elgendy IY, Huo T, Chik V, et al. Efficacy and safety of angiotensin receptor blockers in older patients: a meta-analysis of randomized trials. Am J Hypertens 2015;28(5):576–85.
56. Clegg A, Young J, Iliffe S, et al. Frailty in elderly people. Lancet 2013;381(9868): 752–62.
57. Bally M, Dendukuri N, Rich B, et al. Risk of acute myocardial infarction with NSAIDs in real world use: bayesian meta-analysis of individual patient data. BMJ 2017;357:j1909.

Preoperative Screening

Julianna G. Marwell, MD[a], Mitchell T. Heflin, MD, MHS[b],
Shelley R. McDonald, DO, PhD[b],*

KEYWORDS

- Preoperative evaluation • Function • Morbidity and mortality

KEY POINTS

- Geriatric factors, such as function, mobility, and cognition, predict postoperative morbidity and mortality.
- A geriatric preoperative risk assessment includes detailed evaluations of function, mobility, cognition, medical conditions, and medications.
- Preparation for surgery in older adults requires a detailed discussion to share expected outcomes and risks and gain an understanding of the patient's goals of care.

INTRODUCTION

Approximately one-third of inpatient surgeries performed in the United States occur in adults older than 65.[1,2] Studies have demonstrated that this population has a higher risk of postoperative morbidity and mortality compared with younger patients.[3] Preoperative evaluation provides not only an opportunity to estimate risk, but also an opportunity for health optimization.[4,5] Furthermore, accounting for the broader context of aging and health in the perioperative period can improve identification of goals of care and shared decision making before surgery.[6] The American College of Surgeons National Surgical Quality Improvement Program (ACS NSQIP) and the American Geriatrics Society (AGS) published best practice guidelines to help guide geriatric perioperative care teams in improving both patient outcomes and experience.[7] This article details important aspects of the preoperative assessment related to older adults.

GERIATRIC-FOCUSED PREOPERATIVE ASSESSMENT
Functional Status and Frailty

Measuring function provides critical information about the impact of illness, risk for complications, and needs for adaptive interventions. Functional assessment should

Disclosure Statement: Dr M.T. Heflin is a chapter author for Up to Date, Inc. Drs M.T. Heflin and S.R. McDonald are supported by a grant from the Veterans Administration Office of Academic Affiliations for a Specialty Care Education Center of Excellence.
[a] Department of Medicine, Medical University of South Carolina, 171 Ashley Avenue, Charleston, SC 29425, USA; [b] Division of Geriatrics, Duke University School of Medicine, DUMC Box 3003, Durham, NC 27710, USA
* Corresponding author.
E-mail address: shelley.mcdonald@duke.edu

Clin Geriatr Med 34 (2018) 95–105
https://doi.org/10.1016/j.cger.2017.08.004
0749-0690/18/Published by Elsevier Inc.

be part of the preoperative evaluation for all older adults undergoing complex surgeries, because dependence in even 1 activity of daily living (ADL) is independently associated with increased mortality 30 days after surgery.[8] Moreover, for those undergoing major cardiac surgery, impairment in instrumental ADLs (IADLs) may predict the risk of death at 6 months following the surgery.[9] The ACS NSQIP/AGS Best Practice Guidelines recommends evaluating function using the 4-question Short Simple Screening Test for Functional Assessment:

1. *Can you get out of bed or chair yourself?*
2. Can you dress and bathe yourself?
3. Can you make your own meals?
4. Can you do your own shopping?

A negative response to any of these questions triggers a full inquiry about ADLs and IADLs to identify areas that need to be addressed both before and after surgery.[5]

Frailty, the loss of resilience with increased vulnerability to stressors, is independently associated with greater risk for postoperative complications, increased length of hospital stay, and greater likelihood of being discharged being dependent for care.[10,11] Assessing selected components of frailty, such as gait speed, is more practical than trying to assess frailty as a whole. Slower gait speed alone predicts those at higher risk of postoperative complications. Gait speed less than 0.8 m/s independently predicts poor in-hospital outcomes in those undergoing cardiac surgery.[12,13] The Timed Up and Go (TUG) test measures global functional mobility by having patients rise from a standard chair, walk 10 feet, turn and return to the chair, and sit down. Difficulty standing, or overall time more than 15 seconds predicts falls and should prompt a preoperative physical therapy referral. Although the TUG is the preferred test for falls risk, gait speed may be more informative for those with intermediate walking speeds because each 0.1-m/s decrease in gait speed confers an 11% relative increase in mortality in the setting of cardiac surgery.[13,14]

Robust social support can compensate for losses of both physical and cognitive abilities and improve transitions after surgery. Patients after hip surgery with greater social support had improved functional recovery after 6 months, highlighting the importance of support networks in postoperative outcomes.[15,16]

Cognition

Cognitive impairment is underrecognized in older adults and has important implications for function and health in the perioperative period.[17] First, recognizing underlying cognitive impairment may lead the health care provider to reach out to the patient's family members or caregivers for additional history. Second, meaningful consent requires an understanding of the cognitive abilities. Third, underlying cognitive impairment substantially increases risk for postoperative delirium, which can prolong hospital length of stay and increase morbidity, mortality,[18,19] and postoperative functional impairment.[20] Among older adults with cognitive impairment, proactive measures to mitigate delirium risk can reduce its incidence significantly.[21] Finally, measures of a patient's baseline cognitive function can inform planning for postoperative and postacute care and the need for more social support.

In those without memory concerns, the Mini-Cog[22] effectively assesses for short-term recall and executive function. A more detailed cognitive assessment can be done by using the Montreal Cognitive Assessment (MoCA)[23] or the St Louis University Mental Status Examination (SLUMS).[24]

Sensory

Hearing and vision impairments are increasingly more common with advanced age. Identifying these potential deficits in older adults preoperatively is extremely important, as they are modifiable risk factors for delirium. When addressed as part of a comprehensive risk mitigation plan, the incidence of delirium may be reduced by as much as 40%.[25] Thus, all older adults should be advised to bring their glasses and hearing aids when hospital admission is anticipated.

Mental Health

An emerging body of evidence suggests that mental health disorders are associated with adverse postoperative outcomes in older adults. Patients with depressive symptoms have an increased risk of postoperative delirium and longer length of stay.[26,27] Use of the Geriatric Depression Screen or the Patient Health Questionnaire identifies those at risk for depression.[28] Anxiety, similarly, can have adverse effects on perioperative mental and physical health and is associated with longer lengths of stay.[29,30] Patients with posttraumatic stress disorder (PTSD) appear to be at risk for emergence delirium, which is defined as fearful, aggressive, agitated behaviors that occur immediately following surgery on awakening from anesthetic agents.

Identification of depression, anxiety, and PTSD should trigger nonpharmacologic interventions in the preoperative period, including education/reassurance about the procedure and plans for anesthesia and pain management, instruction in stress reduction techniques, or less traditional approaches, like music and massage.[31] Alcohol abuse and dependence is frequently overlooked in older adults and is associated with increased postoperative complications; therefore, all older adults should be screened for alcohol and substance abuse preoperatively.[32,33]

Medication Management

One in 3 older adults takes 5 or more prescription medications and, as a result, has a high risk of adverse drug events in the perioperative period.[34] Performance of a careful medication review, with particular attention to indication, dose, adverse events, and adherence, identifies inappropriate or incorrectly dosed medications. As medication changes are recommended in the preoperative period, care should be taken to verify the patient's understanding, with strategies such as teach back, and to ensure that they have a reliable system for medication administration.

Certain high-risk situations and medication classes deserve special attention in the perioperative period (Table 1). A general review for other high-risk medications can help identify those that may contribute to postoperative complications. Specifically, medications with anticholinergic properties increase risk of delirium, constipation, urinary retention, and falls. The Anticholinergic Cognitive Burden Scale can help identify these medications to allow for tapering and discontinuation.[35] Additionally, the AGS maintains the Beers Criteria List of potentially inappropriate medications that have an increased risk of adverse effects in older adults.[36]

Pain Management

A comprehensive pain management plan in the preoperative setting may improve postoperative experience and outcomes for older adults. Preoperative assessment should include documentation of current pain character, location, level and functional impact, pharmacologic and nonpharmacologic strategies for management, prior experience with postoperative pain and adverse medication effects, and expectations for the upcoming surgery.[40] In particular, a careful accounting of pain unrelated to the

Table 1
High-risk medications in the perioperative period

Medication Classes	Perioperative Risks	Management Strategy
• Antihypertensives • Diuretics	Hypotension increases risk of MI, stroke, AKI, and death[37]	• Check orthostatic BP and HR and renal function • Hold or reduce dose of medications as indicated • Gradually reintroduce medications postoperatively
• Insulin • Oral hypoglycemic agents	Hypoglycemia	• Assess glucose control and avoid hypoglycemia • Hold hypoglycemics in the immediate perioperative period and manage blood glucose with short-acting insulin until able to maintain oral caloric intake[38]
• Antiplatelet agents • Anticoagulants	Excessive postoperative bleeding, risk of thrombosis	• Assess strength of indication, need for bridging, safety of continuing antiplatelet agents[39] • Consult with specialty providers, including cardiology, neurology, hematology
• Benzodiazepines • Other sedative hypnotics	Delirium, falls, slowed recovery, withdrawal	• Assess chronicity and pattern of use • Consider trial of slow taper if adequate preoperative interval available • Carefully document and communicate clear directions for dosing in the postoperative period • Provide nonpharmacologic approaches for anxiety and insomnia

Abbreviations: AKI, acute kidney injury; BP, blood pressure; HR, heart rate; MI, myocardial infarction.

surgical problem may help planning for recovery. Older patients and their families should have a clear idea of the steps taken to achieve acceptable pain control, including multimodal pharmacologic and nonpharmacologic strategies.

Cardiovascular Risk Stratification

Major adverse cardiac events are a common and lethal complication following major noncardiac surgery among older adults. Rates of postoperative myocardial infarction, congestive heart failure, and stroke increase twofold among those older than age 65 and are associated with higher in-hospital mortality.[41]

Preoperative assessment in older patients begins with risk stratification using validated tools that account for surgery type, cardiac history, functional status, and cardiovascular risk factors. The Revised Cardiac Risk Index is the simplest and most widely used tool, but lacks a measure of function. The NSQIP Myocardial Infarction and Cardiac Arrest Risk Index includes age, functional dependence, American Society of Anesthesiologists (ASA) class and renal impairment (creatinine >1.5 mg/dL) and has an online calculator.[42] Both tools provide estimates of postoperative cardiac morbidity and mortality, which can then inform discussions regarding the risks and benefits of a given surgery. Although electrocardiograms are performed in most preoperative assessments, their use should be reserved for those having intermediate or high-risk surgery, or any patient with known cardiovascular or pulmonary disease or major risk factors. Point-of-care tests for cardiac biomarkers, including B-type natriuretic peptide and troponin provide an additional tool for preoperative cardiac testing,[43] particularly for older adults in whom it may be difficult to assess metabolic equivalents.

Perioperative management of cardioprotective medications requires careful consideration in older adults. Use of beta blockers has been associated with increased risk of stroke and death. As a result, most guidelines now recommend against initiating beta blockers in the perioperative period, particularly if not given adequate time to titrate doses safely. Recent trials offer differing views regarding continuation of aspirin before noncardiac surgery. Most guidelines recommend continuation of aspirin in patients who have a history of cardiovascular disease.[44] However, among those having surgery in a "noncompressible" space (ie, eye, spine, brain, prostate), surgeons will often prefer to stop aspirin 1 week before surgery.

Pulmonary Risk Assessment

Assessing for the risk of postoperative pulmonary complications (PPCs) is important because PPCs are more common than cardiac complications and result in greater in-hospital mortality and probability of being discharged to a skilled nursing facility.[45,46] Predictors of PPCs in older adults include functional dependence, dyspnea, severe chronic obstructive pulmonary disease, low preoperative oxygen saturation, recent respiratory infection, and smoking status. Other factors used for estimating PPCs are age and surgery-related. Advancing age is directly related to risk for PPCs because, unlike cardiac complications, PPCs increase with each decade after age 50, especially for those older than 80.[45] Surgery site is another important factor, as PPCs occur in 2% to 12% of nonthoracic surgeries and up to 38% of thoracic surgeries. Surgeries more than 3 hours in duration predict PPCs. Tools, such as the Assess Respiratory Risk in Surgical Patients in Catalonia (ARISCAT), is an easily administered risk index using 7 objective factors to stratify patients' risk for PPCs.[47] Respiratory muscle training is one strategy to maximize respiratory support in preparation for upcoming surgery that may be particularly beneficial for high-risk surgeries, as it reduces the risk of postoperative atelectasis and pneumonia.[48] Smoking cessation is another modifiable preoperative risk factor that has some mixed evidence and uncertainty about the optimal time period to quit smoking before surgery, but smoking cessation 4 to 8 weeks before surgery appears to reduce postoperative morbidity with longer periods being more beneficial.[49,50] Older studies suggested smoking cessation shortly before surgery contributed to PPC, but more recent meta-analyses and systematic reviews show that smoking cessation within 8 weeks of surgery is not associated with increased PPCs.[51]

Obstructive Sleep Apnea

Obstructive sleep apnea (OSA) increases in prevalence with older age.[52,53] As many as 41% of those undergoing elective surgery may have OSA, and we recommend using a screening tool such as the STOP-BANG questionnaire to help identify those at risk of complications including hypoxemia, pneumonia, respiratory failure, low blood pressure, reduced blood flow to the heart, and atrial fibrillation.[54] All patients should be screened so that the decision can be made to either refer for sleep studies or to minimize aggravating factors, such as anesthetic agents, opioid pain medications, and sedative hypnotics. Screening preoperatively can alert the surgical team to

Table 2
Selected surgical risk prediction models

Risk Calculator Name	Risk Evaluated	Components of Risk	Benefits	Challenges
American College of Surgeons National Surgical Quality Improvement Program (ACS NSQIP)[55]	Death, overall complication, individual complications, readmission, return to OR, discharge to nursing or rehabilitation facility	Age, sex, functional status, emergency, ASA class, chronic steroid use, ascites, sepsis, ventilator dependence, disseminated cancer, diabetes, hypertension, congestive heart failure, dyspnea, smoker within 1 y, severe COPD, dialysis, acute renal failure, BMI	• Provides percentage risk and graphic display	• Need specific procedure name or CPT code
American Society Anesthesiologists (ASA) Class	6 categories of physical health	Level of systemic disease	• Easy to use • Predictor of inpatient mortality[56]	• Highly subjective • Does not account for age, multimorbidity, and complexity of surgery
Hopkins Frailty Index[10,57]	Complications, readmissions, functional dependence	Shrinking (weight loss >10 lb in 1 year), grip strength, exhaustion, low activity, walking speed	• Strong predictive capacity	• Data collection and interpretation can be complex and time consuming
Elderly Physiologic and Operative Severity Score for the enumeration of mortality and morbidity (E-POSSUM)[58]	Postoperative morbidity and mortality	Physiologic: age, cardiac status, respiratory status, ECG, systolic blood pressure, pulse rate, hemoglobin, white blood cell count, blood urea nitrogen, sodium, potassium, Glasgow Coma Scale Operative: operation severity, blood loss, peritoneal contamination, malignancy status, urgency	• Specific for older adults	• Includes intraoperative factors so cannot be calculated preoperatively • Developed on patients receiving colorectal surgery

Abbreviations: ACS, American College of Surgeons; BMI, body mass index; COPD, chronic obstructive pulmonary disease; CPT, current procedural terminology; ECG, electrocardiogram.

potential interventions, such as nocturnal oximetry, semi-upright positioning, and continuous positive airway pressure if tolerated.

DISCUSSION: RISK ASSESSMENT AND SHARED DECISION MAKING

Surgical risk assessment traditionally focuses on morbidity, including the likelihood of common complications, and mortality. Older patients, however, may want more information related to the risk of loss of cognitive and physical function and discharge care needs and location. A variety of risk-prediction models exist with varying degrees of complexity. Several risk-prediction models are listed in **Table 2**.

Determination of risk should lead to discussions with patients regarding their goals and preferences. Many elective surgical procedures, such as knee replacements or cataract removal, are performed to improve quality of life. In the setting of the patient's underlying conditions assessed at the geriatric-focused preoperative visit, realistic outcomes and potential cognitive and functional effects need to be discussed. One study showed that patients and their families need the aforementioned information to make decisions to have surgery.[6] Given that context, a shared decision should be facilitated using tools such as a Question Prompt List to help engage patients in discussions about whether to proceed with such surgery, and if so, then what can be done preoperatively to reduce such risks.[6]

Table 3	
Screening domains for adults older than 65 having elective surgery	
Domain	**Instruments and Inquiry**
Goal setting	• Overall health goals • Patient's understanding of surgery • Provide Question Prompt List
Function and social support	• Short Simple Screening Test ○ If positive, then do full ADLs and IADLs • Social support: current and planned after surgery
Nutrition	• BMI<23 or weight loss of >10% within 6 mo ○ If yes, then do a full assessment with Short Mini-Nutritional Assessment
Mobility	• Gait speed: high risk if <0.8 m/s • Get up and Go: high risk if >15 s
Cognition	• Mini-Cog ○ If positive, then MoCA or SLUMS
Mental health	• Patient Health Questionnaire (PHQ)-2 ○ If positive, then PHQ-9 • Ask about PTSD and anxiety
Medication management	• Detailed medication review • Special focus on high-risk medication classes
Medical conditions	• Cardiac: NSQIP MI and Cardiac Arrest Risk Index • Pulmonary: ARISCAT • Obstructive Sleep Apnea: STOP-BANG
Shared decision making	• Reference QPL • NSQIP Risk Calculator • Communicate plan with surgeon and PCP

Abbreviations: ADL, activity of daily living; ARISCAT, Assess Respiratory Risk in Surgical Patients in Catalonia; BMI, body mass index; IADL, instrumental ADL; MI, myocardial infarction; MoCA, Montreal Cognitive Assessment; NSQIP, National Surgical Quality Improvement Program; PCP, primary care provider; PTSD, posttraumatic stress disorder; QPL, Question Prompt List; SLUMS, St Louis University Mental Status Examination.

SUMMARY

As the number of older adults going for surgical procedures continues to rise, is important to do a geriatric-focused preoperative evaluation with a standard workflow using familiar screening tools. **Table 3** is a framework to guide systematic evaluation for the most complex and vulnerable older adults preparing for surgery.

REFERENCES

1. Sandra L, Colby JMO. Projections of the size and composition of the U.S. population: 2014 to 2060. Current Population Reports, P25–1143. Washington, DC: US Census Bureau; 2015.
2. DeFrances CJ, Lucas CA, Buie VC, et al. National hospital discharge survey. Natl Health Stat Rep 2006;2008(5):1–20.
3. Polanczyk CA, Marcantonio E, Goldman L, et al. Impact of age on perioperative complications and length of stay in patients undergoing noncardiac surgery. Ann Intern Med 2001;134(8):637–43.
4. Kim KI, Park KH, Koo KH, et al. Comprehensive geriatric assessment can predict postoperative morbidity and mortality in elderly patients undergoing elective surgery. Arch Gerontol Geriatr 2013;56(3):507–12.
5. Chow WB, Rosenthal RA, Merkow RP, et al. Optimal preoperative assessment of the geriatric surgical patient: a best practices guideline from the American College of Surgeons national surgical quality improvement program and the American Geriatrics Society. J Am Coll Surgeons 2012;215(4):453–66.
6. Steffens NM, Tucholka JL, Nabozny MJ, et al. Engaging patients, health care professionals, and community members to improve preoperative decision making for older adults facing high-risk surgery. JAMA Surg 2016;151(10):938–45.
7. Mohanty S, Rosenthal RA, Russell MM, et al. Optimal perioperative management of the geriatric patient: a best practices guideline from the American College of Surgeons NSQIP and the American Geriatrics Society. J Am Coll Surgeons 2016;222(5):930–47.
8. Scarborough JE, Bennett KM, Englum BR, et al. The impact of functional dependency on outcomes after complex general and vascular surgery. Ann Surg 2015;261(3):432–7.
9. Kim DH, Kim CA, Placide S, et al. Preoperative frailty assessment and outcomes at 6 months or later in older adults undergoing cardiac surgical procedures: a systematic review. Ann Intern Med 2016;165(9):650–60.
10. Makary MA, Segev DL, Pronovost PJ, et al. Frailty as a predictor of surgical outcomes in older patients. J Am Coll Surgeons 2010;210(6):901–8.
11. Robinson TN, Wu DS, Pointer L, et al. Simple frailty score predicts postoperative complications across surgical specialties. Am J Surg 2013;206(4):544–50.
12. Afilalo J, Eisenberg MJ, Morin JF, et al. Gait speed as an incremental predictor of mortality and major morbidity in elderly patients undergoing cardiac surgery. J Am Coll Cardiol 2010;56(20):1668–76.
13. Afilalo J, Kim S, O'Brien S, et al. Gait speed and operative mortality in older adults following cardiac surgery. JAMA Cardiol 2016;1(3):314–21.
14. Viccaro LJ, Perera S, Studenski SA. Is timed up and go better than gait speed in predicting health, function, and falls in older adults? J Am Geriatr Soc 2011;59(5):887–92.
15. Ayers DC, Franklin PD, Ring DC. The role of emotional health in functional outcomes after orthopaedic surgery: extending the biopsychosocial model to orthopaedics: AOA critical issues. J Bone Joint Surg Am 2013;95(21):e165.

16. Cummings SR, Phillips SL, Wheat ME, et al. Recovery of function after hip fracture the role of social supports. J Am Geriatr Soc 1988;36(9):801–6.

17. Culley DJ, Flaherty D, Reddy S, et al. Preoperative cognitive stratification of older elective surgical patients: a cross-sectional study. Anesth analgesia 2016;123(1): 186–92.

18. Robinson TN, Wu DS, Pointer LF, et al. Preoperative cognitive dysfunction is related to adverse postoperative outcomes in the elderly. J Am Coll Surgeons 2012;215(1):12–7 [discussion: 17–8].

19. Witlox J, Eurelings LM, de Jonghe JM, et al. Delirium in elderly patients and the risk of postdischarge mortality, institutionalization, and dementia: a meta-analysis. JAMA 2010;304(4):443–51.

20. Quinlan N, Rudolph JL. Postoperative delirium and functional decline after noncardiac surgery. J Am Geriatr Soc 2011;59(Suppl 2):S301–4.

21. Marcantonio ER, Flacker JM, Wright RJ, et al. Reducing delirium after hip fracture: a randomized trial. J Am Geriatr Soc 2001;49(5):516–22.

22. Borson S, Scanlan JM, Chen P, et al. The mini cog as a screen for dementia: validation in a population based sample. J Am Geriatr Soc 2003;51(10):1451–4.

23. Nasreddine ZS, Phillips NA, Bédirian V, et al. The Montreal Cognitive Assessment, MoCA: a brief screening tool for mild cognitive impairment. J Am Geriatr Soc 2005;53(4):695–9.

24. Tariq SH, Tumosa N, Chibnall JT, et al. Comparison of the Saint Louis University Mental Status Examination and the Mini-Mental State Examination for detecting dementia and mild neurocognitive disorder—a pilot study. Am J Geriatr Psychiatry 2006;14(11):900–10.

25. Inouye SK, Bogardus ST Jr, Charpentier PA, et al. A multicomponent intervention to prevent delirium in hospitalized older patients. New Engl J Med 1999;340(9): 669–76.

26. Smith PJ, Attix DK, Weldon BC, et al. Depressive symptoms and risk of postoperative delirium. Am J Geriatr Psychiatry 2016;24(3):232–8.

27. Taylor WD. Clinical practice. Depression in the elderly. New Engl J Med 2014; 371(13):1228–36.

28. Siu AL, Bibbins-Domingo K, Grossman DC, et al. Screening for depression in adults: US preventive services task force recommendation statement. JAMA 2016;315(4):380–7.

29. Williams JB, Alexander KP, Morin JF, et al. Preoperative anxiety as a predictor of mortality and major morbidity in patients aged >70 years undergoing cardiac surgery. Am J Cardiol 2013;111(1):137–42.

30. Poole L, Leigh E, Kidd T, et al. The combined association of depression and socioeconomic status with length of post-operative hospital stay following coronary artery bypass graft surgery: data from a prospective cohort study. J Psychosomatic Res 2014;76(1):34–40.

31. Wilson CJ, Mitchelson AJ, Tzeng TH, et al. Caring for the surgically anxious patient: a review of the interventions and a guide to optimizing surgical outcomes. Am J Surg 2016;212(1):151–9.

32. Blazer DG, Wu LT. The epidemiology of at-risk and binge drinking among middle-aged and elderly community adults: national survey on drug use and health. Am J Psychiatry 2009;166(10):1162–9.

33. Nath B, Li Y, Carroll JE, et al. Alcohol exposure as a risk factor for adverse outcomes in elective surgery. J Gastrointest Surg 2010;14(11):1732–41.

34. Hewitt J, McCormack C, Tay HS, et al. Prevalence of multimorbidity and its association with outcomes in older emergency general surgical patients: an observational study. BMJ Open 2016;6(3):e010126.
35. Salahudeen MS, Duffull SB, Nishtala PS. Anticholinergic burden quantified by anticholinergic risk scales and adverse outcomes in older people: a systematic review. BMC Geriatr 2015;15:31.
36. By the American Geriatrics Society 2015 Beers Criteria Update Expert Panel. American Geriatrics Society 2015 updated Beers criteria for potentially inappropriate medication use in older adults. J Am Geriatr Soc 2015;63(11):2227–46.
37. Walsh M, Devereaux PJ, Garg AX, et al. Relationship between intraoperative mean arterial pressure and clinical outcomes after noncardiac surgery: toward an empirical definition of hypotension. Anesthesiology 2013;119(3):507–15.
38. Dhatariya K, Levy N, Kilvert A, et al. NHS diabetes guideline for the perioperative management of the adult patient with diabetes. Diabetic Med 2012;29(4):420–33.
39. Douketis JD, Spyropoulos AC, Kaatz S, et al. Perioperative bridging anticoagulation in patients with atrial fibrillation. New Engl J Med 2015;373(9):823–33.
40. Chou R, Gordon DB, Leon-Casasola OA, et al. Management of postoperative pain: a clinical practice guideline from the American Pain Society, the American Society of Regional Anesthesia and Pain Medicine, and the American Society of Anesthesiologists' Committee on Regional Anesthesia, Executive Committee, and Administrative Council. J Pain 2016;17(2):131–57.
41. Davenport DL, Ferraris VA, Hosokawa P, et al. Multivariable predictors of postoperative cardiac adverse events after general and vascular surgery: results from the patient safety in surgery study. J Am Coll Surgeons 2007;204(6):1199–210.
42. Gupta PK, Gupta H, Sundaram A, et al. Development and validation of a risk calculator for prediction of cardiac risk after surgery. Circulation 2011;124(4): 381–7.
43. Devereaux P, Sessler DI. Cardiac complications in patients undergoing major noncardiac surgery. New Engl J Med 2015;373(23):2258–69.
44. Goldhammer JE, Herman CR, Sun JZ. Perioperative aspirin in cardiac and noncardiac surgery. J Cardiothorac Vasc Anesth 2017;31(3):1060–70.
45. Pfeifer KJ, Smetana GW. Pulmonary risk assessment and optimization. Hospital Medicine Clinics 2016;5(2):176–88.
46. Friedman SM, Mendelson DA, Kates SL, et al. Geriatric co-management of proximal femur fractures: total quality management and protocol-driven care result in better outcomes for a frail patient population. J Am Geriatr Soc 2008;56(7): 1349–56.
47. Canet J, Gallart L, Gomar C, et al. Prediction of postoperative pulmonary complications in a population-based surgical cohort. Anesthesiology 2010;113(6): 1338–50.
48. Katsura M, Kuriyama A, Takeshima T, et al. Preoperative inspiratory muscle training for postoperative pulmonary complications in adults undergoing cardiac and major abdominal surgery. Cochrane Database Syst Rev 2015;(10):CD010356.
49. Thomsen T, Villebro N, Møller AM. Interventions for preoperative smoking cessation. Cochrane Database Syst Rev 2000;7:CD002294.
50. Mills E, Eyawo O, Lockhart I, et al. Smoking cessation reduces postoperative complications: a systematic review and meta-analysis. Am J Med 2011;124(2): 144–54.e8.
51. Myers K, Hajek P, Hinds C, et al. Stopping smoking shortly before surgery and postoperative complications: a systematic review and meta-analysis. Arch Intern Med 2011;171(11):983–9.

52. Young T, Peppard PE, Taheri S. Excess weight and sleep-disordered breathing. J Appl Physiol (1985) 2005;99(4):1592–9.
53. Hoch CC, Reynolds CF 3rd, Monk TH, et al. Comparison of sleep-disordered breathing among healthy elderly in the seventh, eighth, and ninth decades of life. Sleep 1990;13(6):502–11.
54. Vasu TS, Doghramji K, Cavallazzi R, et al. Obstructive sleep apnea syndrome and postoperative complications: clinical use of the STOP-BANG questionnaire. Arch otolaryngol Head Neck Surg 2010;136(10):1020–4.
55. Cologne KG, Keller DS, Liwanag L, et al. Use of the American College of Surgeons NSQIP surgical risk calculator for laparoscopic colectomy: how good is it and how can we improve it? J Am Coll Surgeons 2015;220(3):281–6.
56. Wolters U, Wolf T, Stützer H, et al. ASA classification and perioperative variables as predictors of postoperative outcome. Br J Anaesth 1996;77(2):217–22.
57. Fried LP, Tangen CM, Walston J, et al. Frailty in older adults: evidence for a phenotype. J Gerontol A Biol Sci Med Sci 2001;56(3):M146–57.
58. Tran Ba Loc P, du Montcel ST, Duron JJ, et al. Elderly POSSUM, a dedicated score for prediction of mortality and morbidity after major colorectal surgery in older patients. Br J Surg 2010;97(3):396–403.

Driving Dilemmas
A Guide to Driving Assessment in Primary Care

Emily Morgan, MD

KEYWORDS

- Geriatrics • Driving • Assessment • Safety • Mandatory reporting

KEY POINTS

- Life expectancy exceeds driving fitness expectancy in the United States, meaning most older adults will need to retire from driving in their lifetime.
- Driving safety relies on the coordination of multiple complex functions, including visual acuity and perception; cognitive abilities, including executive function and multitasking; and neuromuscular function.
- There is no single validated screening tool to assess driving safety; thus, evaluation requires a multifaceted approach.
- Primary care providers should know local reporting laws and should be competent to counsel their patients on driving cessation and alternative transportation strategies.

INTRODUCTION

Clinical assessment of driving ability is one of the most challenging problems for those who provide primary care to older adults. In our aging population, older drivers are increasing in number and driving more miles than in the past.[1,2] It is estimated that by 2050, drivers aged 65 years and older will comprise 25% of the US driving population.[3] Although age is not a reliable predictor of driving safety, age-related changes in both physical and cognitive abilities may affect driving safety over time.[4] Around 70 years of age fatal crash rates per mile traveled begin to significantly increase, and fatal crash rates among all drivers are highest for those aged 85 years and older.[3,5]

Some states have passed legislation to tighten license renewal requirements for older drivers, and many others are considering similar options. However, it is important to keep in mind that driving often equates to independence for older adults. Life expectancy in the United States exceeds driving fitness expectancy by roughly 6 years for men and

Disclosure Statement: The author has nothing to disclose.
Division of General Internal Medicine and Geriatrics, Oregon Health and Science University, Mail Code L-475, 3181 South West Sam Jackson Park Road, Portland, OR 97239, USA
E-mail address: morganem@ohsu.edu

10 years for women.[2] When older adults are forced to stop driving, they depend on others for transportation and may be at risk for social isolation and increased rates of depression and anxiety.[6–8] For these reasons, appropriate and accurate assessment of fitness to drive is key to both safety and quality of life in older adults.

Studies looking at self-rated driving ability show that older drivers tend to score themselves higher on ability as their skills decline.[9] At the same time, studies looking at driving cessation show that older drivers feel strongly about making their own decisions regarding driving.[10] However, most older adults agree that if a primary care provider advised them to stop driving, they would do so.[11] Given this dichotomy between driving perception and ability, it is clearly within the role of primary care providers to assess and counsel older drivers and to make recommendations or referrals as necessary. The goal of this review is to give primary care providers an overview of appropriate driver assessment and provide tools to accomplish this as efficiently as possible in a busy primary care setting.

WHEN TO ASSESS FOR DRIVING FITNESS

Driving safety is not a reflection of age, but ability; there are no guidelines on when to screen for driving ability. Studies of driving patterns among older drivers show stronger associations between cessation of driving and impairment in visual, motor, and cognitive functions than with any specific diagnosis.[2,7] This finding makes knowing when to screen for driving impairment difficult; it falls to patients, families, and the provider to pay attention to warning signs of declining ability. Acute events, such as hospitalizations, or acute worsening of chronic conditions should alert providers to assess driving safety.[12] **Box 1**

Box 1
Red flag conditions to prompt driver assessment

History of falls

Gait impairment

Peripheral neuropathy

Orthostatic hypotension

Syncope or presyncope

Stroke or TIA

Seizure

Recurrent hypoglycemia

Visual impairment despite correction

Vertigo

Neurodegenerative diseases (eg, Parkinson, MS, SCA)

Cognitive impairment

Functional impairment in ADLs or IADLs

Delirium

Alcohol or substance abuse

Chronic use of high-risk medications

Abbreviations: ADLs, activities of daily living; IADLs, instrumental activities of daily living; MS, multiple sclerosis; SCA, spinocerebellar ataxia; TIA, transient ischemic attack.

lists clinical conditions that increase the risk of driving impairment and warrant initiating driving assessment. Note, these red flag conditions do not automatically indicate the inability to drive safely but should act as a prompt for further inquiry about driving safety.

In addition to the review of risky clinical conditions, medication review is an important piece of driving assessment. There are many prescription and nonprescription medications that can potentially impair driving.[12] The most common medications that increase the risk of driving impairment can be found in **Box 2**. For older adults who are currently on medications who are concerning for driving safety, clinicians should engage in risk-benefit discussions regarding the taper or discontinuation of medications versus voluntary cessation of driving. Although there will be many times that a risky medication can be tapered or discontinued, there will also be times when the benefit of the medication outweighs the risks associated with driving cessation. In these cases, it is the clinician's responsibility to inform patients of the risks of driving impairment; some states may require mandatory reporting if the medication is continued.[13]

Along with the discussion of medications and driving, providers should talk with older adults about alcohol and substance use. Data from the National Survey on Drug Use and Health Report in 2014 estimated that 4.1% of drivers older than 65 years drove under the influence of alcohol in the preceding year. That is roughly the same percentage as drivers aged 16 to 17 years.[14] Although clinicians may not think to assess for alcohol abuse in older adults, repeated studies have shown the prevalence of at-risk drinking (drinking 5 or more drinks in 1 day) in this age group ranges from 2% to 10%.[15] Although substance use is risky for any driver, older adults are at an even greater risk because of the increased rates of drug interactions, decreased alcohol metabolism, and underlying cognitive impairment.[15] The US Preventive Services Task Force recommends screening all adults for alcohol misuse on an annual basis; if older patients are found to have at-risk drinking, a review of driving safety is warranted.

Even when patients present without red flag medical conditions, medication lists, or substance issues, driving concerns should be a part of a geriatric review of systems during annual examinations. Asking 2 simple questions (Do you have any concerns about driving or limit your driving in any way? Has anyone else expressed concern about your driving?) can bring to light driving issues that would otherwise go undetected. If patients or families report accidents, traffic tickets, getting lost, or driving limited to a time of day or location, a driving assessment should be completed.

Box 2
High-risk medications for driver impairment
Anticholinergics
Anticonvulsants
Benzodiazepines
Opiates
Parkinson medications
Hypnotics
Antipsychotics
Muscle relaxants
Stimulants
Antidepressants

DRIVER ASSESSMENT

There is no single validated screening instrument for driver safety[16]; but once a clinician has detected a red flag condition, medication, or positive review of systems, an office-based driving assessment should be completed. The 3 main components of driver assessment include vision assessment, cognitive assessment, and neuromuscular function assessment.[12,16,17]

VISION ASSESSMENT

Visual acuity and perception are paramount to driver ability. As people age, visual deficits become increasingly common because of conditions such as cataracts, retinopathy, glaucoma, and macular degeneration. These conditions do not just reduce acuity but can also cause poor depth perception and limit peripheral vision, which are associated with decreased ability to judge distance and speed.[18] In one recent study on crashes involving older drivers, inadequate surveillance described as the driver looking but not seeing a roadway hazard was the most common form of driver error.[19]

Visual acuity and visual fields can be easily tested in the office. Acuity, as measured by a Snellen chart, should be tested with patients' usual eyewear at a distance of 20 ft first with both eyes, then with each eye individually. Visual acuity requirements vary state to state and range from 20/40 to 20/70; but if acuity is less than 20/40, referral to ophthalmology is warranted.[16] If visual fields are abnormal by confrontation testing in each eye, the referral to ophthalmology should specifically request visual fields testing with perimetry.

COGNITIVE ASSESSMENT

Several cognitive domains are necessary for safe driving. These domains include short-term and working memory, visual processing, attention, multitasking, planning, and executive function.[12,20] It is important to remember that a diagnosis of mild cognitive impairment or even early dementia does not automatically mean that patients are not safe to drive. On the flip side of this coin, it is equally important to remember that not all patients without a diagnosis of dementia are fit to drive. Traffic accidents involving older adults are most often caused by errors of recognition, which are errors caused by distractibility, inability to multitask, and decreased visual processing.[19] Attention and multitasking are frontal lobe functions that are known to decrease with age in healthy brains, starting around the fifth decade of life.[21] This decrease is due to age-related white matter changes that are seen in normal aging brains.[22] Although most older drivers are fit to drive, detecting deficits in attention and multitasking, even in patients with normal cognitive function, will help detect those whose impairments are significant enough to need to stop driving.

The most recommended cognitive tests for driving ability are the clock draw and the Trail Making Test (TMT).[12,16,20,23–25] These tests should be administered individually for patients without known cognitive impairment.[26] The TMT has 2 parts (A and B), and it is part B that measures working memory and the ability to shift attention and has been shown to be more closely associated with driving outcomes. Although impairments in clock draw and TMT are predictive of poor driving skill, it is important to remember that neither is sensitive or specific enough in patients without dementia to revoke a driving license but should prompt an on-the-road driving test.

For patients with known cognitive impairment, these tests can be administered together as part of the Montreal Cognitive Assessment (MoCA, available at mocatest.org).[27] Those with a MoCA score of 18 out of 30 or less are likely unsafe to drive (75% sensitivity, 94% specificity). Although driving may be safe in early dementia, patients should be reassessed every 6 to 12 months.[28] Patients with confirmed moderate to severe dementia should no longer be allowed to drive based on multiple published guidelines.[28]

NEUROMUSCULAR FUNCTION

Driving is a physical activity as much as it is a cognitive one. Flexibility, proprioception, coordination, and adequate reaction time are all required for safe driving.[12,26] On average, a driver will need to make 20 major decisions for each mile driven and has roughly 0.5 second to respond in order to avoid a potential accident.[29] Clearly, assessment of neuromuscular function is imperative to ensure safe driving.

Just as we see cognitive changes in healthy older adults, we see a decline in motor function with normal aging.[30] Motor deficits are seen across motor domains with age, including gait and balance, sensorimotor adaptation, motor sequencing, and motor control.[30,31] We also see a reduction in muscle strength with aging. After 70 years of age, muscle strength decreases roughly 3% per year.[32] Flexibility of the neck and trunk are also reduced with age, which can lead to the inability to assess the road adequately.[33] Movement may also be limited by pain due to age-related disease, such as osteoarthritis.[12]

All neuromuscular changes seen in aging make driving a potential hazard. Slower reaction times can make it difficult to respond to stimuli appropriately, such as identifying a gap between cars and being able to appropriately enter the flow of traffic at the right time and speed.[34] One study found that a history of falls was associated with motor vehicle accidents in which older drivers were found to be at fault.[35] Other studies have shown driving impairment to be associated with the inability to reach above the shoulder, impaired left knee flexion, and the inability to walk for more than one block.[36,37]

Several motor and flexibility tests have been studied in traffic research,[26] but few have been readily adapted to primary care settings. Recommended clinical assessments include thorough neurologic and musculoskeletal examinations, paying special attention to range of motion and motor strength, as well as a test of gait speed.[12,26] In a recent review, the Timed Up and Go test was not a reliable indicator of driving ability[38] but the rapid-pace walk test was associated with driving ability.[16] The rapid-pace walk test is performed by timing patients while they walk a total of 20 ft (10 ft up and back) using any assistive device they normally use. Completion of the test in greater than 9 seconds is associated with driving impairment.[39]

WHAT TO DO WHEN AN OLDER ADULT IS DEEMED TO BE AN AT-RISK DRIVER

Once red flag conditions have been identified and office-based driver assessment has been completed, the next step is to differentiate between conditions that are mild, controllable, or reversible and those that are severe, uncontrollable, or permanent (**Fig. 1**). Patients with moderate to severe dementia or permanent uncontrollable disease states that prevent safe driving should be counseled to give up driving immediately and may need to be reported to the Department of Motor Vehicles (DMV) depending on local laws.[28] However, many patients have conditions that would benefit from interventions that may result in improved driving ability.

Workup and treatment of reversible causes of disease is always the first step in addressing driver safety. Interventions, such as changing medications to lower-risk regimens or referral to ophthalmology for appropriate eyewear or cataract removal, can lower the driving risk.[12] Referral to physical or occupational therapy may be

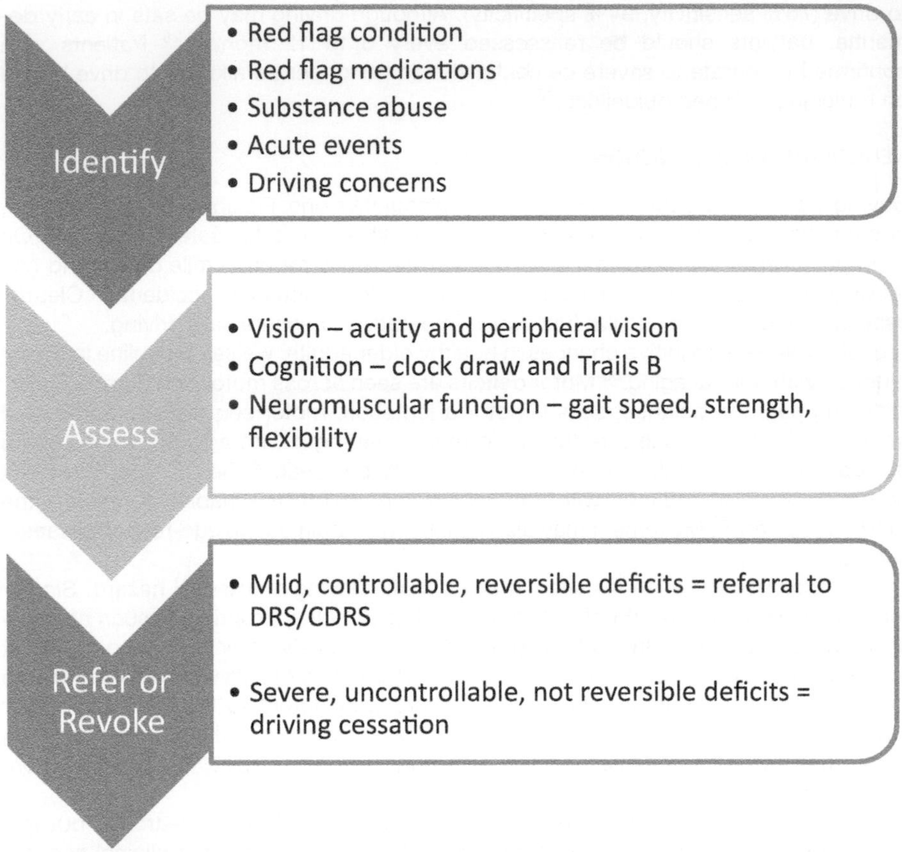

Identify
- Red flag condition
- Red flag medications
- Substance abuse
- Acute events
- Driving concerns

Assess
- Vision – acuity and peripheral vision
- Cognition – clock draw and Trails B
- Neuromuscular function – gait speed, strength, flexibility

Refer or Revoke
- Mild, controllable, reversible deficits = referral to DRS/CDRS
- Severe, uncontrollable, not reversible deficits = driving cessation

Fig. 1. Driver assessment workflow. CDRS, certified driver rehabilitation specialists; DRS, driver rehabilitation specialists.

appropriate for those patients whose neuromuscular or cognitive deficits are potentially reversible.

For patients with impairments not easily identified as reversible and not severe enough to warrant immediate revocation of driving privileges, the gold standard is on-the-road driving assessment with specially trained driver rehabilitation specialists (DRS) or certified DRS (CDRS). These providers are trained in functional assessment, including vehicle safety and mobility, environmental awareness, adherence to traffic laws, and reaction time. They can offer strategies to improve driver safety, such as the use of adaptive equipment or driver safety courses. They will also advise patients to stop driving if significant improvements are not achievable.

Providers should be aware that not all DRS and CDRS offer on-the-road assessment or rehabilitation services. Patients should be directed toward the most comprehensive services available to avoid the need for multiple referrals. Driving assessment is also not routinely covered by insurance, and patients should be warned of out-of-pocket costs ranging from $200 to $400 for assessment and $100/h for rehabilitation services.[12] If driving assessment is not available or feasible, referral to your local DMV is often the best choice.

If driving cessation is advised, providers should be prepared to counsel patients on alternative transportation strategies. Reviewing support systems, identifying barriers, and providing patients a list of local resources can prevent social isolation. Providers should also plan to follow up with patients regarding mood, as depression and anxiety increase in prevalence in older adults who have had to give up driving.[6]

DRIVING LAWS

The current laws regarding older drivers vary by state. In some states, older drivers are required to renew their licenses more frequently. Other states require frequent vision testing or do not allow renewal by mail. In Illinois, drivers older than 75 years are required to perform a road test at renewal, whereas the District of Columbia requires physician approval for drivers older than 70 years. Licensing departments have the right to revoke or restrict a license if the driver is found to be impaired. Restrictions may include nighttime or highway driving.[13]

Requirements for DMV referral also vary by state, and some states require providers to fill out paperwork before an on-the-road driving evaluation will be considered. In some states, primary care providers are mandatory reporters, which makes them vulnerable to both civil and criminal liability for not reporting unsafe drivers. The Health Insurance Portability and Accountability Act (HIPPA) laws allow for reporting protected health information when it is in the public interest; thus, reporting to the DMV is allowed within privacy laws. It is recommended that all providers familiarize themselves with the reporting laws in their state and to document thoroughly all discussions and assessments related to driving.

SUMMARY

Clinical assessment of driving ability remains a challenging but necessary part of primary care practice. Knowing most people will need to retire from driving during their lifetimes, it is important to feel comfortable assessing and counseling older adults about driving. This overview of appropriate driver assessment offers tools to effectively and efficiently assess driver safety using evidence-based strategies, including visual, neuromuscular, and cognitive assessments, and offers guidance on when to refer to rehab services or to revoke driving privileges.

REFERENCES

1. National Center for Injury Prevention and Control. Web-based injury statistics query and reporting system (WISQARS), 2014 fatal injury data. Atlanta (GA): Centers for Disease Control and Prevention; 2015. Available at: http://www.cdc.gov/injury/wisqars/index.html. Accessed April 10, 2017.
2. Foley DJ, Heimovitz HK, Guralnik JM, et al. Driving life expectancy of persons aged 70 years and older in the United States. Am J Public Health 2002;92(8): 1284–9.
3. Traffic Safety Facts 2013. A compilation of motor vehicle crash data from the fatality analysis reporting system and the general estimates system National Highway Traffic Safety Administration National Center for Statistics and Analysis U.S. Department of Transportation. Washington, DC. Available at: https://crashstats.nhtsa.dot.gov/Api/Public/ViewPublication/812139. Accessed March 18, 2017.
4. Anstey KJ, Wood J, Lord S, et al. Cognitive, sensory and physical factors enabling driving safety in older adults. Clin Psychol Rev 2005;25:45–65.
5. Cicchino JB. Why have fatality rates among older drivers declined? The relative contributions of changes in survivability and crash involvement. Accid Anal Prev 2015;83:67–73.

6. Fonda SJ, Wallace RB, Herzog AR. Changes in driving patterns and worsening depressive symptoms among older adults. J Gerontol B Psychol Sci Soc Sci 2001;56:343–51.

7. Marottoli RA, Ostfeld AM, Merrill SS, et al. Driving cessation and changes in mileage driven among elderly individuals. J Gerontol 1993;48:255–60.

8. Liddle J, Gustafsson L, Mitchell G, et al. A difficult journey: reflections on driving and driving cessation from a team of clinical researchers. Gerontologist 2017; 57(1):82–8.

9. Freund B, Colgrove LA, Burke BL, et al. Self-rated driving performance among elderly drivers referred for driving evaluation. Accid Anal Prev 2005 Jul;37(4): 613–8.

10. Choi M, Mezuk B, Rebok G. Voluntary and involuntary driving cessation in later life. J Gerontological Social Work 2012;55(4):367–76.

11. Betz M, Schwartz R, Valley M, et al. Older adult opinions about driving cessation: a role for advanced driving directives. J Prim Care Community Health 2012;3(3): 150–4.

12. Clinician's guide to assessing and counseling older drivers. Third edition 2015: an update of the physician's guide to assessing and counseling older drivers. Available at: https://www.nhtsa.gov/.../nti/older_drivers/.../812228_CliniciansGuideToOlderDrivers.pdf. Accessed April 30, 2017.

13. Older drivers: license renewal procedures. Insurance Institute for Highway Safety 2013. Available at: http://www.iihs.org/iihs/topics/laws/olderdrivers?topicName=older-drivers. Accessed March 12, 2017.

14. Lipari R, Hughes A, Bose J. Driving under the influence of alcohol and illicit drugs. The CBHSQ report. Rockville (MD): Substance Abuse and Mental Health Services Administration (US); 2016. Available at: https://www.ncbi.nlm.nih.gov/books/NBK424784/. Accessed March 12, 2017.

15. Barry KL, Blow FC. Drinking across the life span: focus on older adults. Alcohol Res 2016;38(1):115–20.

16. Dickerson AE, Meuel DB, Ridenour CD, et al. Assessment tools predicting fitness to drive in older adults: a systematic review. Am J Occup Ther 2014;68(6): 670–80.

17. Desapriya E, Subzwari S, Fujiwara T, et al. Conventional vision screening tests and older driver motor vehicle crash prevention. Int J Inj Contr Saf Promot 2008;15(2):124–6.

18. West CG, Gildengorin G, Haegerstrom-Portnoy G, et al. Vision and driving self-restriction in older adults. J Am Geriatr Soc 2003;51:1348–55.

19. Cicchino JB. Critical older driver error in a national sample of serious U.S. crashes. Accid Anal Prev 2015;80:211–9.

20. Asimakopulos J, Boychuck Z, Sondergaard D, et al. Assessing executive function in relation to fitness to drive: a review of tools and their ability to predict safe driving. Aust Occup Ther J 2012;59:402–27.

21. Reuter-Lorenz G, Cabeza R, Dennis N. Frontal lobes and aging: deterioration and compensation. In: principles of frontal lobe function. Oxford (United Kingdom): Oxford University Press; 2013.

22. Costello MC, Madden DJ, Mitroff SR, et al. Age-related decline of visual processing components in change detection. Psychol Aging 2010;25:356–68.

23. Vanlaar W, McKiernan A, McAteer H, et al. A meta-analysis of cognitive screening tools for drivers aged 80 and over. Ottawa (Canada): Traffic injury research foundation; 2014. Available at: http://tirf.ca/wpcontent/uploads/2017/01/MTO_cognitive_meta_6.pdf. Accessed on April 23, 2017.

24. Seong-Youl C, Jae-Shin L, A-Young S. Cognitive test to forecast unsafe driving in older drivers: meta-analysis. NeuroRehabilitation 2014;35(4):771–8.

25. Papndonatos GD, Ott BR, Barco PP, et al. Clinical utility of the trail-making test as a predictor of driving performance in older adults. J Am Geriatr Soc 2015;63(11): 2358–64.

26. Karthaus M, Falkenstein M. Functional changes and driving performance in older drivers: assessment and interventions. Geriatrics 2016;1(2):12.

27. Hollis AM, Duncanson H, Kapust LR, et al. Validity of the Mini-Mental State Examination and the Montreal Cognitive Assessment in the prediction of driving test outcome. J Am Geriatr Soc 2015;63:988–92.

28. Cameron D, Zucchero-Sarracini C, Rozmovits L, et al. Development of a decision-making tool for reporting drivers with mild dementia and mild cognitive impairment to transportation administrators. Int Psychogeriatr 2017;29(9):1551–63.

29. American Automobile Association. Senior driving: understand mind and body changes 2017. Available at: http://seniordriving.aaa.com/understanding-mind-body-changes/reaction-time. Accessed April 23, 2017.

30. Bernard JA, Seidler RD. Moving forward: age effects on the cerebellum underlie cognitive and motor declines. Neurosci Biobehavioral Rev 2014;42:193–207.

31. Boisgontier MP. Motor aging results from cerebellar neuron death. Trends Neurosciences 2015;38:127–8.

32. Clark BC, Taylor JL. Age-related changes in motor cortical properties and voluntary activation of skeletal muscle. Curr Aging Sci 2011;4(3):192–9.

33. Chen KB, Xu X, Lin JH, et al. Evaluation of older driver head functional range of motion using portable immersive virtual reality. Exp Gerontol 2015;70:150–6.

34. Der G, Deary IJ. Age and sex differences in reaction time in adulthood: results from the United Kingdom Health and Lifestyle Survey. Psychol Aging 2006;21: 62–73.

35. Huisingh C, McGwin G, Orman KA, et al. Frequent falling and motor vehicle collision involvement in older drivers. J Am Geriatr Soc 2014;62:123–9.

36. Hu Hu PS, Trumble DA, Foley DJ, et al. Crash risks of older drivers: a panel data analysis. Accid Anal Prev 1998;30:569–81.

37. Marottoli RA, Wagner DR, Cooney LM, et al. Predictors of crashes and moving violations among elderly drivers. Ann Intern Med 1994;121:842–6.

38. Mielenz TJ, Durbin LL, Cisewski JA, et al. Select physical performance measures and driving outcomes in older adults. Inj Epidemiol 2017;4(1):14.

39. Staplin L, Gish KW, Wagner EK. MaryPODS revisited: updated crash analysis and implications for screening program implementation. J Saf Res 2003;34:389–97.

Prevention and Screening of Unhealthy Substance Use by Older Adults

Benjamin H. Han, MD, MPH[a],*, Alison A. Moore, MD, MPH[b]

KEYWORDS

- Older adults • Substance use • Screening tools • Prevention • Assessment tools

KEY POINTS

- Unhealthy alcohol use and illegal drug use among older adults is increasing dramatically with the aging of the Baby Boomer Generation.
- Substance use disorders are a chronic and often relapsing brain disease that may be difficult to recognize in older adults.
- Owing to the physiologic changes of aging, concurrent chronic medical diseases, and high use of prescription medications, older adults are at high risk for adverse effects of alcohol and illegal drugs.
- When screening and discussing substance use with older adults it is important to use nonjudgmental and nonstigmatizing language.

INTRODUCTION

Historically, older adults have not had high rates of substance use and, previously, older adults reduced their substance use with increasing age.[1] However, this is changing considerably with the aging population and the large Baby Boomer generation, who have higher reported rates of substance use compared with any preceding generation, and changing attitudes toward alcohol and recreational use of illegal drugs.[2–4] Therefore, the rates of substance use by older adults and the number at risk for its unhealthy use will increase.

Unhealthy substance use is typically defined as the use of alcohol more than guideline-recommended levels[5] or the use of tobacco products, illegal drugs, or the nonmedical use of prescription drugs (use for the feeling or experience or taking

Disclosure Statement: The authors have no disclosures.
[a] Division of Geriatric Medicine and Palliative Care, Department of Medicine, New York University School of Medicine, 550 First Avenue, BCD 615, New York, NY 10016, USA; [b] Department of Medicine, University of California, San Diego School of Medicine, 9500 Gilman Drive, La Jolla, CA 92093, USA
* Corresponding author.
E-mail address: Benjamin.Han@nyumc.org

more than prescribed), and includes the full range of harmful use and substance use disorders (SUDs).[6] Based on the *Diagnostic and Statistical Manual of Mental Disorders, 5th edition* (DSM-5), the diagnosis of SUDs is established by a pattern of use that causes clinically significant functional impairment (**Table 1**).[7] The DSM-5 brought notable changes in the nomenclature of SUDs with the elimination of the terms substance abuse and dependence.

Substance use may have important health impacts, especially among older adults who are at higher risk for chronic diseases and who often take more medications than younger adults. Adults with SUDs have higher hospitalization rates, and acute health care costs, in comparison with the general population.[8] Given the possible negative impacts of alcohol and drug use on chronic diseases and drug–medication interactions among an aging population, screening and prevention of unhealthy substance use is critical to address the potential enormous public health impact of increasing substance use by older adults.

PREVALENCE OF USE AND HEALTH-RELATED RISKS OF ALCOHOL, TOBACCO, AND OTHER DRUGS
Alcohol Use

Unhealthy alcohol use is common, and alcohol accounts for one of the leading causes of preventable death in the United States.[9] Alcohol remains the most commonly used substance among older adults, and is expected to continue to increase considerably.[4] The 2013/2014 National Survey on Drug Use and Health (NSDUH) estimated the prevalence for alcohol use within the past year among older adults to be 62.1%, with rates of binge drinking to be 21.5% in older men and 9.1% in older women, and alcohol use disorders were estimated to be 5.1% in men and 2.4% in women.[10] These national estimates represent dramatic increases from 2005 and 2006, with a 19.2% relative increase in binge drinking and 23.3% relative increase in alcohol use disorders among older adults.[10]

Although there is evidence that moderate alcohol use (usually ≤1 drink daily) may be associated with decreases in morbidity and mortality among older adults,[3,11] the risk of mortality increases with heavier drinking.[11] There are physiologic changes that occur with aging that place older adults at higher risk for adverse outcomes including diminished liver function, decreases in total body water, and neuronal sensitivity to alcohol, which increases sensitivity and decreases tolerance of alcohol.[12] In addition, alcohol can cause or exacerbate medical conditions in older adults such as hypertension, arrhythmias, hemorrhagic stroke, cirrhosis, gastrointestinal bleeding, and certain cancers.[13] This makes older adults particularly vulnerable to the negative effects of alcohol, particularly when drinking in excess of recommended drinking limits.[14] In addition, prescribed medications have the potential to interact with alcohol, and can lead to adverse effects.[15] Specifically, binge drinking may be particularly harmful for older adults and may increase the risk for unintentional injuries (ie, falls) and negatively impact existing chronic diseases.[16,17]

Owing to these vulnerabilities, the National Institute on Alcohol Abuse and Alcoholism recommends a lower threshold for recommended drinking limits for both older men and women. For older adults (>65 years of age) who are healthy and do not take medications the recommended guidelines include no more than 3 drinks on a given day and no more than 7 drinks in 1 week (**Box 1**).[17] Proposals have been made to lower the recommended drinking limits based on comorbidities for older adults.[15] However, many older adults and their providers may not be aware of the National Institute on Alcohol Abuse and Alcoholism lower drinking

Table 1
SUD criteria

DSM-5 Criteria for SUD	Considerations for the Older Adult
A substance is often taken in larger amounts or over a longer period than was intended.	Cognitive impairment can prevent adequate self-monitoring. Substances themselves may more greatly impair cognition among older adults than younger adults.
There is a persistent desire or unsuccessful efforts to cut down or control substance use.	It is the same as the general adult population.
A great deal of time is spent in activities necessary to obtain the substance, use the substance, or recover from its effects.	Consequences from substance use can occur from using relatively small amounts.
There is craving or a strong desire to use the substance.	It is the same as the general adult population. Older adults with entrenched habits may not recognize cravings in the same way as the general adult population.
There is recurrent substance use resulting in a failure to fulfill major role obligations at work, school, or home.	Role obligations may not exist for older adults in the same way as for younger adults because of life stage transitions, such as retirement. The role obligations more common in late life are caregiving for an ill spouse or family member, such as a grandchild.
There is continued substance use despite having persistent or recurrent social or interpersonal problems caused or exacerbated by the effects of the substance.	Older adults may not realize the problems they experience are from substance use.
Important social, occupational, or recreational activities are given up or reduced because of substance use.	Older adults may engage in fewer activities regardless of substance use, making it difficult to detect.
There is recurrent substance use in situations in which it is physically hazardous.	Older adults may not identify or understand that their use is hazardous, especially when using substances in smaller amounts.
Substance use is continued despite knowledge of having a persistent or recurrent physical or psychological problem that is likely to have been caused or exacerbated by the substance.	Older adults may not realize the problems they experience are from substance use.
Tolerance is developed, as defined by either of the following: 1. A need for markedly increased amounts of the substance to achieve intoxication or the desired effect; or 2. A markedly diminished effect with continued use of the same amount of the substance.	Because of the increased sensitivity to substances as they age, older adults will seem to have lowered rather than increase in tolerance.

(continued on next page)

Table 1 (continued)	
DSM-5 Criteria for SUD	**Considerations for the Older Adult**
Withdrawal, as manifested by either of the following: 1. The characteristic withdrawal syndrome for the substance; or 2. The substance or a close relative is taken to relieve or avoid withdrawal symptoms.	Withdrawal symptoms can manifest in ways that are more "subtle and protracted." Late-onset substance users may not develop physiologic dependence; or nonproblematic users of medications, such as benzodiazepines, may develop physiologic dependence.

Substance use disorder (SUD, formerly substance abuse or dependence) is defined as a medical disorder in which 2 or more of the listed symptoms are occurring in the last 12 mo.

Adapted from Barry KL, Blow FC, Oslin DW. Substance abuse in older adults: review and recommendations for education and practice in medical settings. Subst Abuse 2002;23(Suppl 3):105–31; and *Data from* American Psychiatric Association. Diagnostic and statistical manual of mental disorders. 5th edition. Arlington (VA): American Psychiatric Publishing; 2013. p. 491; and *From* Kuerbis A, Sacco P, Blazer D, et al. Substance abuse among older adults. Clin Geriatr Med 2014;30:629–54; with permission.

recommended guidelines for older adults, and continue to drinking at potentially unhealthy levels as they age.

Tobacco Use

An estimated 8.4% of adults 65 and older are current smokers.[18] Unlike alcohol, there are no possible health benefits of smoking, and its health risks particularly for cardiovascular and pulmonary systems along with the increased risk for malignancy and mortality are all well-documented.[19] For older adults, smoking has been associated with cognitive decline,[20] functional limitations,[21] and places older adults at a higher risk for geriatric conditions.[22] Although most older smokers have attempted unsuccessfully to quit on multiple occassions,[23] the benefits of smoking cessation are clear at any age. Many studies have confirmed that quitting smoking, even after the age of 65, results in significantly reduced mortality compared with those who continue to smoke.[24]

Box 1
National Institute on Alcohol Abuse and Alcoholism guidelines for alcohol use for older adults

1. Healthy adults over the age of 65 who do not take medications should not consume more than:
   - 7 standard drinks per week,
     Or
   - 3 standard drinks on any given day.

2. A standard drink is defined as:
   - One 12-ounce can or bottle of regular beer, ale, or wine cooler;
   - One 8- or 9-ounce can or bottle of malt liquor;
   - One 5-ounce glass of red or white wine; or
   - One 1.5-ounce shot glass of distilled spirits (gin, rum, tequila, vodka, whiskey, etc). The label on the bottle will say 80 proof or less.

Adapted from the National Institute on Alcohol Abuse and Alcoholism (NIAAA). Older Adults and Alcohol. Rockville (MD): NIAAAA; 2015. Available at: https://pubs.niaaa.nih.gov/publications/olderAdults/olderAdults.htm. Accessed June 5, 2017.

Illegal Drug Use

The same physiologic changes with aging that increase the effect of alcohol in older adults also increase the effect of other drugs including benzodiazepines, opioids, and marijuana. With widespread changes in attitudes toward marijuana, its legalization for recreational use in several states, and its increasing use for medicinal purposes, marijuana use is more prevalent than other "illicit" drugs among older adults.[25,26] The NSDUH estimated a national prevalence of past-year marijuana use in 2012 and 2013 of 4.8% among older adults with a 57.8% relative increase from 2006 and 2007 among adults aged 50 to 64 and a 250% relative increase among adults 65 and older.[25] Although marijuana and its cannabis formulations may be useful as a medical treatment for seizures, multiple sclerosis, chronic pain, and other chronic conditions,[27] research into its benefits are limited, and the risks of marijuana for older adults are largely unknown. Some evidence suggests that marijuana's effect on increasing the heart rate may increase the risk for cardiovascular disease and that smoking marijuana may also increase the risk for lung disease and infections.[27] Marijuana has been linked with an increased risk of cerebrovascular events,[28] may have significant drug–drug interactions,[27] and there are concerns about its effects on short-term and long-term cognitive funcitoning.[29] Future studies are needed to help providers balance the potential risks and benefits of marijuana use among older adults, particularly among those with multiple chronic conditions and high prescription medication use.

The use of other illicit drugs besides marijuana remains low among older adults in the general population.[2,3] Although only 0.41% of adults 50 and older reported past year use of cocaine in the 2005 and 2006 NSDUH,[2] other studies done in inner-city hospital settings show a substantially higher prevalence of cocaine use among older adults ranging from 2% to 2.3%.[30,31] Older adults may be particularly vulnerable to the adverse effects of cocaine use, particularly on the cardiovascular and cerebrovascular[32] systems that can lead to disability or sudden death. Similarly, although the NSDUH estimated the prevalence of past-year heroin use by older adults to be 0.03%, in certain populations there is a higher prevalence; for example, New York City has seen dramatic increases in opioid treatment program use by older adults for problems with heroin use.[33]

Prescription Drug Misuse

Older adults widely use medications, as one US representative study found among adults 62 to 85 years of age, at least 87% used at least one prescription medication and 36% used 5 or more.[34] This places older adults at increasing risk for drug-drug interactions and misuse, and 1 study found at least 1 in 4 older adults use psychoactive medications with misuse potential.[35] The result has been dramatic increases in emergency department visits involving prescription misuse by adults 50 and older (an increase of 121% from 2004 to 2008) with pain relievers and medications for anxiety or insomnia being the most common culprits.[36]

This increase has been occurring in the setting of the quadrupling of prescription opioid analgesics in the last decade, particularly among older adults.[37] An estimated 1.4% of adults aged 50 and over used prescription opioids nonmedically in the past year.[2] Older adults are at particularly high risk for opioid overdose and older adults with opioid use disorders are at risk for greater mortality.[38] Further study is needed to better understand the impact of chronic opioid use on chronic conditions, functional status, and health care use among older adults. The other medication often prescribed to older adults with high misuse potential are benzodiazepines. Despite well-documented risks of benzodiazepines in older adults, which include falls, cognitive impairment, delirium, fatigue, and potential adverse interactions with prescribed medications,[39] benzodiazepines continue to be widely prescribed to older adults with rates as high as 30% in some populations.[40,41] Providers need to be aware that, for older adults, benzodiazepines should never be used as a first-line treatment for agitation or insomnia, and that long-acting benzodiazepines should never be used for any indication by older adults.[42]

PREVENTION AND SCREENING
Prevention

The prevention of unhealthy substance use and SUDs includes abstinence and reductions in the amount of substance use. Although there is scant evidence regarding universal prevention programs targeted for older adults to abstain or reduce substance use, some health education programs have been shown to increase knowledge regarding unhealthy alcohol use among older adults.[43,44] In the setting of the prescription opioid epidemic, careful prescribing practices can help prevent prescription drug misuse. Providers need to be aware of a patient's history of unhealthy alcohol or drug use, and try to avoid prescribing drugs that can place patients at an increased risk for misuse or relapse.[45] In addition, prescription drug monitoring programs[46] and online training programs in managing chronic pain and opiate prescribing (including the Centers for Disease Control and Prevention's Guideline for Prescribing Opioids for Chronic Pain,[47] available at: https://www.cdc.gov/drugoverdose/prescribing/guideline.html) are useful tools to help providers practice safe prescribing and prevent prescription drug misuse. The need for scientific research in nonaddictive treatments for chronic pain is a priority at the National Institutes of Health.[48]

Screening

Despite the increasing prevalence of unhealthy substance use among older adults, they are less likely to be screened for unhealthy substance use compared with younger adults.[3] Screening for substance use faces many barriers, including lack of time and the challenges of integrating screening into regular clinical workflow both in primary care and in the inpatient setting.[49,50] In addition, both patients and providers may be uncomfortable discussing and reporting stigmatized behavior, such as substance use.[51] Also, the similarities of the signs and symptoms of substance use may be mistaken for manifestations of other chronic diseases, and a common perception among older adults is that symptoms of substance use are related to aging or other diseases and not to the substance itself.[3] Regardless of its difficulties, universal screening will help to identify patients who may be at risk for or are currently engaging in unhealthy substance use behaviors.

Approach to screening

When assessing individuals of any age regarding substance use, it is vital to understand that stigma is a major barrier for people with SUDs from seeking and receiving help.[52] Therefore, it is imperative that the language used when discussing issues of substance use with patients does not further stigmatize. In 2016, The White House Office of National Drug Control Policy released guidance on the importance of language surrounding addiction.[53] In general, it recommended to use the more medically accurate terminology of "substance use disorder," "unhealthy use," or "harmful use" and remove stigmatizing language such as "addict," "abuser," and "addicts."[53,54] This may be especially important when talking with older adults, who have lived through the punitive language surrounding the "war on drugs" and may be particularly sensitive to the use of such stigmatizing language, and therefore not as forthcoming with problems with substance use.

Scientific evidence shows that SUDs are a chronic brain disease, often with periods of recurrence, and a strong genetic component that can produce profound changes in the brain structure and function.[53] Thus, it is important that providers talk with patients about substance use in the same way they discuss other chronic medical conditions, such as cardiovascular disease or diabetes. Therefore, the discussion surrounding alcohol and other substance use should take place in the context of an older adult's overall assessment with the goals of improving health, maintaining function and independence, and improving quality of life.

When screening older adults for unhealthy substance use, it is also important to recognize that specific biologic and social factors unique to older adults may pose challenges in the accurate diagnosis of SUDs. **Table 1** presents several DSM-5 criteria for SUDs and list special considerations for older adults. Many of the DSM-5 criteria may not be relevant to many older adults owing to changes in role obligations or social isolation, or physiologic changes of aging that affect tolerance to certain drugs.[3]

Screening tools

Several screening instruments for substance use are available for a range of substances (alcohol, tobacco, illicit drugs, and prescription drugs), but only a handful were designed specifically for and validated in older adults. Interview-administered 1-item and 2-item screening tests for unhealthy alcohol and other drug use have been validated in the general population, and may be a way to initiate asking about substance use (**Box 2**).[55–57] An alternative are self-administered screening tools, which may help patients to feel more comfortable reporting stigmatized behavior. One example is the Substance Use Brief Screen, which is a self-administered brief screener for tobacco, alcohol, and drug use (illegal and prescription) that has been validated in the primary care setting.[58] A negative screen on the 1-item and 2-item screening tests or a self-administered screener would indicate that screening is complete and allows the provider to provide reinforcement of healthy use patterns related to substance use. Screening positive would lead to further screening with longer, but more reliable screening instruments.

Box 2
One-item and 2-item screening tests for alcohol and/or other drug misuse for older adults

Single-question screening test for unhealthy alcohol use[56]:
   Question: "How many times in the past year have you had 4 or more drinks in a day?"
   Response: A response of greater than 1 is positive.

Single-question screening test for drug use[57]:
   Question: "How many times in the past year have you used an illegal drug or used a prescription medication for nonmedical reasons?"
   Response: A response of 1 or more is positive.

Two-item conjoint screen for alcohol and other drug problems[58]:
   Questions: "In the last year, have you ever drunk or used drugs more than you meant to?"
   "Have you felt you wanted or needed to cut down on your drinking or drug use in the last year?"
   Response: A response of 1 or more is positive for a current substance use disorder.

Adapted from Strobbe S. Prevention and screening, brief intervention, and referral to treatment for substance use in primary care. Prim Care 2014;41(2):189; with permission.

SELECTED SCREENING INSTRUMENTS
The CAGE and CAGE-AID

The CAGE questionnaire[59] is one of the most commonly used screening tools for unhealthy alcohol use and has been studied in older adults with a sensitivity of 86% and a specificity of 78% to detect lifetime alcohol use disorders.[60] The limitations of the CAGE is that it does poorly in identifying binge drinkers[61] and does not distinguish between lifetime or current use.

The Michigan Alcohol Screening Test—Geriatric Version

The Michigan Alcohol Screening Test—Geriatric Version (MAST-G)[62] is the first instrument specifically designed to identify drinking problems among older adults. The MAST-G has 24 yes/no questions with 5 or more positive responses indicating problematic alcohol use. The questions focus more on potential stressors and behaviors that are common among older adults. The MAST-G has high sensitivity (95%) and specificity (78%), and generally has strong psychometric properties.[63]

The Alcohol Use Disorders Identification Test

The Alcohol Use Disorders Identification Test (AUDIT)[64] was developed by the World Health Organization as a screening tool to assess for excessive drinking. The AUDIT has been used in a variety of settings and diverse populations, including older adults.[65] The AUDIT contains 10 items that assess for alcohol consumption, drinking behaviors, and alcohol-related problems in the past year.

The Alcohol, Smoking, and Substance Involvement Screening Test

The Alcohol, Smoking, and Substance Involvement Screening Test is another screening instrument developed by the World Health Organization that screens across all substances including tobacco, alcohol, and illegal drug use.[66] It is an interview-administered screen with 8 questions that help to assess the level of risk for the previous 3 months and can guide treatment decisions. The Alcohol, Smoking, and Substance Involvement Screening Test, although widely used in research and clinical practice, has not yet been validated in older adults.[3]

The Comorbidity—Alcohol Risk Evaluation Tool

The Comorbidity—Alcohol Risk Evaluation Tool[67] is a screening instrument for alcohol use that identifies older adults with specific health behaviors and risks that place them at increased risk for harm from alcohol. It has been validated in older adults with a high sensitivity (92%), but with a lower specificity (51%), mainly owing to most older adults being identified as at risk given their use of medications.[67]

ASSESSMENT, BRIEF INTERVENTION, AND REFERRAL TO TREATMENT

Following the steps in the National Institute on Alcohol Abuse and Alcoholism and the National Institute on Drug Abuse recommendations, when the initial screening of an older individual indicates they are engaging in unhealthy substance use, it is recommended that clinicians share their findings and make clear recommendations. For example, a provider might say, "Based on your responses to the screening questions, your current use is more than is medically safe." It is important to relate the advice about substance use to the patient's overall health, and using nonjudgmental, nonstigmatizing language. This is an opportunity for providers to deliver a brief intervention that engages the patient in education about the substance, its potential health-related consequences, providing feedback, and advice. It is also an opportunity to share how guidelines specifically relate to older adults, and how substances may adversely impact other chronic diseases. Brief interventions provide the older adult with information about potential harms and consequences of substance use, attempt to enhance motivation to change, and, where needed, refer to more intensive services. Brief interventions that focus on alcohol and prescription medication misuse have been found to be effective for older adults.[68] Brief interventions can vary in length from 15 minutes to 1 hour sessions, can be performed in almost any clinical setting, and by almost any trained medical staff.

Older adults identified as needing more treatment than brief interventions can deliver should be referred to specialty treatment. The Substance Abuse and Mental Health Services Administration (SAMHSA) Substance Abuse Treatment Services Locator lists and provides information about state-licensed substance use treatment facilities throughout the United States, which currently number more than 11,000. Treatment options specifically tailored for older adults are beyond the scope of this article, but unfortunately are limited and is an area that needs more active research.[3] Screening, Brief Intervention, and Referral to Treatment for substance use is a nationwide, evidence-based, public health approach initiative funded through the SAMHSA.[69] Screening, Brief Intervention, and Referral to Treatment has been implemented in a variety of settings, and has been adapted for older adults by SAMHSA-funded projects,[70] and has the potential to reach the increasing population of older adults who may engage in unhealthy substance use.

SUMMARY

Alcohol, tobacco, and SUDs are a major public health issue contributing to a devastating increase in overdose mortality, health care costs, and suffering for individuals and their communities. It is important to recognize that the number of older adults who engage in unhealthy substance use is increasing dramatically, and presents unique challenges for prevention and screening. There are unique physiologic and social changes with aging that need to be considered in screening older adults for unhealthy substance use behaviors, and providers need to be mindful the language used when talking about substance use and SUDs with their older patients. Finally, the potential harms of substance use in the setting of an increase in chronic medical diseases, geriatric conditions, and medication use needs to be better understood, and should be an area of priority in research.

REFERENCES

1. Moore AA, Kuerbis A, Dattoma L, et al. Unhealthy substance use in older adults. In: Busby-Whitehead J, editor. Reichel's care of the elderly: clinical aspects of aging. 7th edition. New York: Cambridge University Press; 2016. p. 285–97.
2. Blazer DG, Wu L. The epidemiology of substance use and disorders among middle aged and elderly community adults: National Survey on Drug Use and Health. Am J Geriatr Psychiatry 2009;17:237–45.
3. Kuerbis A, Sacco P, Blazer D, et al. Substance abuse among older adults. Clin Geriatr Med 2014;30:629–54.
4. Moore AA, Karno MP, Grella CE, et al. Alcohol, tobacco, and nonmedical drug use in older U.S. adults: data from the 2001/02 National Epidemiologic Survey of Alcohol and Related Conditions. J Am Geriatr Soc 2009;57(12):2275–81.
5. National Institute on Alcohol Abuse and Alcoholism. Drinking levels defined. 2016. Available at: https://www.niaaa.nih.gov/alcohol-health/overview-alcohol-consumption/moderate-binge-drinking. Accessed May 5, 2017.

6. American Society of Addiction Medicine. Terminology Related to the Spectrum of Unhealthy Substance Use. 2013. Available at: https://www.asam.org/docs/default-source/public-policy-statements/1-terminology-spectrum-sud-7-13.pdf?sfvrsn=2. Accessed May 5, 2017.

7. American Psychiatric Association. Diagnostic and statistical manual of mental disorders. 5th edition. Arlington (VA): American Psychiatric Publishing; 2013.

8. Gryczynski J, Schwartz RP, O'Grady KE, et al. Understanding patterns of high-cost health care use across different substance user groups. Health Aff 2016; 35(1):12–9.

9. Mokdad AH, Marks JS, Stroup DF, et al. Actual causes of death in the United States, 2000. JAMA 2004;291(10):1238–45.

10. Han BH, Moore AA, Sherman S, et al. Demographic trends of binge alcohol use and alcohol use disorders among older adults in the United States, 2005-2014. Drug Alcohol Depend 2016;170:198–207.

11. Thun MJ, Peto R, Lopez AD, et al. Alcohol consumption and mortality among middle-aged and elderly U.S. adults. N Engl J Med 1997;337(24):1705–14.

12. Kennedy GJ, Efremova I, Frazier A, et al. The emerging problems of alcohol and substance abuse in late life. J Soc Distress Homel 1999;8(4):227–39.

13. Center for Substance Abuse Treatment. Substance abuse among older adults. Rockville (MD): Substance Abuse and Mental Health Services Administration (US); 1998 (Treatment Improvement Protocol (TIP) Series, No. 26.) Chapter 2-Alcohol. Available at: https://www.ncbi.nlm.nih.gov/books/NBK64412/. Accessed May 5, 2017.

14. Moore AA, Giuli L, Gould R, et al. Alcohol use, comorbidity, and mortality. J Am Geriatr Soc 2006;54:757–62.

15. Moore AA, Whiteman EJ, Ward KT. Risks of combined alcohol-medication use in older adults. Am J Geriatr Pharmacother 2007;5:64–74.

16. Centers for Disease Control, 2015. Fact sheets – binge drinking. Available at: http://www.cdc.gov/alcohol/fact-sheets/binge-drinking.htm. Accessed May 5, 2017.

17. National Institute of Alcohol Abuse and Alcoholism. Older adults. Bethesda (MD): NIAAA; 2016. Available at: https://www.niaaa.nih.gov/alcohol-health/special-populations-co-occurring-disorders/older-adults. Accessed May 5, 2017.

18. Centers for Disease Control and Prevention. Current cigarette smoking among adults—United States, 2005–2015. MMWR Morb Mortal Wkly Rep 2016;65(44): 1205–11.

19. Centers for Disease Control and Prevention. Health effects of cigarette smoking. Available at: https://www.cdc.gov/tobacco/data_statistics/fact_sheets/health_effects/effects_cig_smoking. Accessed May 5, 2017.

20. Sabia S, Elbaz A, Dugravot A, et al. Impact of smoking on cognitive decline in early old age the Whitehall II cohort study. Arch Gen Psychiatry 2012;69(6): 627–35.

21. Rapuri PB, Gallagher JC, Smith LM. Smoking is a risk factor for decreased physical performance in elderly women. J Gerontol 2007;62A(1):93–100.

22. Nicita-Mauro V, Balbo CL, Mento A, et al. Smoking, aging and the centenarians. Exp Gerontol 2008;43:95–101.

23. Rimer BK, Orleans CT, Keintz MK, et al. The older smoker. Status, challenges and opportunities for intervention. Chest 1990;97:547–53.

24. Taylor DH Jr, Hasselblad V, Henley SJ, et al. Benefits of smoking cessation for longevity. Am J Public Health 2002;92:990–6.

25. Han BH, Sherman S, Mauro PM, et al. Demographic trends among older cannabis users in the United States, 2006-2013. Addiction 2016;112(3):516–25.
26. Pew Research Center. Majority now supports legalizing cannabis. Available at: http://www.people-press.org/2013/04/04/majority-now-supports-legalizing-marijuana. Accessed May 5, 2017.
27. National Institute on Drug Abuse. DrugFacts: marijuana. Available at: http://www.drugabuse.gov/publications/drugfacts/marijuana. Accessed May 5, 2017.
28. Hackam DG. Cannabis and stroke. Stroke 2015;46:852–6.
29. Grant L, Gonzalez R, Carey CL, et al. Non-acute (residual) neurocognitive effects of cannabis use: a meta-analytic study. J Int Neuropsychol Soc 2003;9:679–89.
30. Chait R, Fahmy S, Caceres J. Cocaine abuse in older adults: an underscreened cohort. J Am Geriatr Soc 2010;58(2):391–2.
31. Rudolf M, Penny B, Jennifer M. Mortality rates and predictors of mortality among late-middle-aged and older substance abuse patients. Alcohol Clin Exp Res 1994;18:187–95.
32. Fustinoni O, Ruggiero HA. Acute cerebrovascular accidents in geriatrics. Medical treatment. Rev Asoc Med Argent 1964;78:176–80.
33. Han B, Polydorou S, Ferris R, et al. Demographic trends of adults in New York city opioid treatment programs - an aging population. Subst Use Misuse 2015;50(13):1660–7.
34. Qato DM, Wilder J, Schumm LP, et al. Changes in prescription and over-the-counter medication and dietary supplement use among older adults in the United States, 2005 vs 2011. JAMA Intern Med 2016;176:473.
35. Simoni-Wastila L, Yang HK. Psychoactive drug abuse in older adults. Am J Geriatr Pharmacother 2006;4:380–94.
36. Substance Abuse and Mental Health Services Administration (SAMHSA). Highlights of the 2010 Drug Abuse Warning Network (DAWN) findings on Drug-Related Emergency Department Visits. 2012. Available at: https://www.samhsa.gov/data/sites/default/files/DAWN096/DAWN096/SR096EDHighlights2010.pdf. Accessed May 5, 2017.
37. Sullivan MD, Howe CQ. Opioid therapy for chronic pain in the US: promises and perils. Pain 2013;154(Suppl 1):S94–100.
38. Larney S, Bohnert AS, Ganoczy D, et al. Mortality among older adults with opioid use disorders in the Veteran's Health Administration, 2000-2011. Drug Alcohol Depend 2015;147:32–7.
39. American Geriatrics Society 2015 Beers Criteria Update Expert Panel. American Geriatrics Society 2015 updated Beers criteria for potentially inappropriate medication use in older adults. J Am Geriatr Soc 2015;63(11):2227–46.
40. Achildi O, Leong SH, Maust DT, et al. Patterns of newly-prescribed benzodiazepines in late life. Am J Geriatr Psychiatry 2013;21(Suppl 1(3)):S90–1.
41. Llorente M, David D, Golden AG, et al. Defining patterns of benzodiazepine use in older adults. J Geriatr Psychiatry Neurol 2000;13:150–60.
42. American Geriatrics Society. Choosing wisely. Revised April 23, 2015. Available at: http://www.choosingwisely.org/clinician-lists/american-geriatrics-society-benzodiazepines-sedative-hypnotics-for-insomnia-in-older-adults. Accessed May 5, 2017.
43. Fink A, Beck JC, Wittrock MC. Informing older adults about nonhazardous, hazardous, and harmful alcohol use. Patient Educ Couns 2001;45(2):133–41.
44. Nguyen K, Fink A, Beck JC, et al. Feasibility of using an alcohol-screening and health education system with older primary care patients. J Am Board Fam Pract 2001;14(1):7–15.

45. Strobbe S. Prevention and screening, brief intervention, and referral to treatment for substance use in primary care. Prim Care 2014;41(2):185–213.

46. US Department of Justice, Drug Enforcement Agency (DEA). State prescription drug monitoring programs. Available at: http://www.deadiversion.usdoj.gov/faq/rx_monitor.htm. Accessed May 5, 2017.

47. Centers for Disease Control and Prevention (CDC). CDC guideline for prescribing opioids for chronic pain. Available at: https://www.cdc.gov/drugoverdose/prescribing/guideline.html. Accessed May 5, 2017.

48. Volkow ND, Collins FS. The role of science in addressing the opioid crisis. N Engl J Med 2017;377(4):391–4.

49. Aira M, Kauhanen J, Larivaara P, et al. Factors influencing inquiry about patients' alcohol consumption by primary health care physicians: qualitative semi-structured interview study. Fam Pract 2003;20(3):270–5.

50. Yoast RA, Wilford BB, Hayashi SW. Encouraging physicians to screen for and intervene in substance use disorders: obstacles and strategies for change. J Addict Dis 2008;27(3):77–97.

51. Tourangeau R, Smith TW. Asking sensitive questions—the impact of data collection mode, question format, and question context. Publ Opin Q 1996;60:275–304.

52. Substance Abuse and Mental Health Services Administration (SAMHSA). Results from the 2012 National Survey on Drug Use and Health: summary of national findings. Rockville (MD): Substance Abuse and Mental Health Services Administration; 2013. NSDUH Series H-46, HHS Publication No. (SMA) 13–4795.

53. Botticelli MP, Koh HK. Changing the language of addiction. JAMA 2016;316(13):1361–2.

54. Kelly JF, Wakeman SE, Saitz R. Stop talking 'dirty': clinicians, language, and quality of care for the leading cause of preventable death in the United States. Am J Med 2015;128(1):8–9.

55. Smith PC, Schmidt SM, Allensworth-Davies D, et al. Primary care validation of a single-question alcohol screening test. J Gen Intern Med 2009;24(7):783–8.

56. Smith PC, Schmidt SM, Allensworth-Davies D, et al. A single-question screening test for drug use in primary care. Arch Intern Med 2010;170(13):1155–60.

57. Brown RL, Leonard T, Saunders LA, et al. A two-item conjoint screen for alcohol and other drug problems. J Am Board Fam Pract 2001;14(2):95–106.

58. McNeely J, Strauss SM, Saitz R, et al. A brief patient self-administered substance use screening tool for primary care: two-site validation study of the Substance Use Brief Screen (SUBS). Am J Med 2015;128(7):784.e9-19.

59. Ewing JA. Detecting alcoholism. The CAGE questionnaire. JAMA 1984;252(14):1905–7.

60. Stewart D, Oslin DW. Recognition and treatment of late-life addictions in medical settings. J Clin Geropsychol 2001;7(2):145–58.

61. Adams W, Barry KL, Fleming MF. Screening for problem drinking in older primary care patients. JAMA 1996;276:1964–7.

62. Blow FC, Brower KJ, Schulenberg JE, et al. The Michigan alcohol screening test: geriatric version (MAST-G): a new elderly specific screening instrument. Alcohol Clin Exp Res 1992;16:172.

63. Blow FC, Gillespie BW, Barry KL, et al. Brief screening for alcohol problems in elderly populations using the Short Michigan Alcoholism Screening Test-Geriatric Version (SMAST-G). Alcohol Clin Exp Res 1998;22(Suppl):131A.

64. Babor TF, Higgins-Biddle JC, Saunders JB, et al. The Alcohol Use Disorders Identification Test (AUDIT): guidelines for use in primary care. 2nd edition.

Geneva (Switzerland): Department of Mental Health and Substance Dependence, World Health Organization; 2001.

65. Beullens J, Aertgeerts B. Screening for alcohol abuse and dependence in older people using DSM criteria: a review. Aging Ment Health 2004;8(1):76–82.

66. Humeniuk R, Henry-Edwards S, Ali R, et al. The alcohol, smoking, and substance involvement screening test (ASSIST). Geneva (Switzerland): World Health Organization; 2010.

67. Moore AA, Beck JC, Babor TF, et al. Beyond alcoholism: identifying older, at-risk drinkers in primary care. J Stud Alcohol 2002;63(3):316–24.

68. Kuerbis A, Sacco P. A review of existing treatments for substance abuse among the elderly and recommendations for future directions. Subst Abuse 2013;7: 13–37.

69. Substance Abuse and Mental Health Services Administration (SAMHSA). Screening, brief intervention, and referral to treatment (SBIRT). Available at: http://www.samhsa.gov/prevention/sbirt. Accessed May 5, 2017.

70. Schonfeld L, Hazlett RW, Hedgecock DK, et al. Screening, brief intervention, and referral to treatment for older adults with substance misuse. Am J Public Health 2015;105(1):205–11.

Vaccinations in Older Adults

Megan Burke, MD[a],*, Theresa Rowe, DO, MS[b]

KEYWORDS

- Vaccinations • Immunizations • Older adults • Immune senescence
- Pneumococcal • Influenza • Herpes zoster

KEY POINTS

- Older adults are at increased risk for vaccine-preventable infections. Rates of immunizations among older adults remain lower than goal despite guidelines, leaving room for intervention and improvement.
- Most of the morbidity and mortality related to vaccine-preventable illnesses in older adults in the United States is related to influenza and pneumococcal disease.
- There is a high-dose influenza vaccination specifically targeted for older adults; however, the Advisory Committee on Immunization Practices does not express preference for either high-dose or standard-dose influenza vaccine use in this population.
- Cost of immunizations influence vaccination rates in older adults.

INTRODUCTION

Vaccines are important for preventing infections in older adults aged ≥65 years. It is estimated that more than 40,000 older adults die each year in the United States from vaccine-preventable infections, with influenza being the largest contributor.[1] Increasing the rate of vaccinations among older adults is a priority of the US government addressed in the Healthy People 2020 initiative.[2] Older adults are at increased risk for serious complications from vaccine-preventable illnesses due to age-associated changes in immune function, and chronic medical comorbidities, which place them at both higher risk for infection and for having an infection with a protracted course.[3] Although practice guidelines are well established by the Advisory Committee on Immunization Practices (ACIP), and endorsed by most professional societies, vaccination rates for older adults remain low, with approximately 74.0% of

Disclosure Statement: No disclosures.
a Geriatric Medicine and Gerontology, Johns Hopkins University School of Medicine, Johns Hopkins Bayview Medical Center, 5200 Eastern Avenue, MFL Center Tower, Suite 2200, Baltimore, MD 21224, USA; b General Internal Medicine and Geriatrics, Northwestern Feinberg School of Medicine, 750 North Lakeshore Drive, 10th Floor, Chicago, IL 60611, USA
* Corresponding author.
E-mail address: mburke31@jhmi.edu

older adults receiving the influenza vaccination during the 2015 influenza season, 64.0% of older adults receiving any pneumococcal vaccination as of 2015, and only 27.9% of eligible older adults reported receiving the herpes zoster vaccine in 2014.[4] This article focuses on the following vaccines recommended for older adults: (1) influenza; (2) pneumococcal; (3) herpes zoster; (4) tetanus, diphtheria, pertussis; and (5) hepatitis, and how cost and public misconceptions influence vaccination rates in this population.

INFLUENZA VACCINATION

Adults aged ≥65 years are at greater risk for serious complications from influenza compared with younger adults because of age-associated changes in immune function.[3] The Centers for Disease Control and Prevention (CDC) estimated that more than 50% of influenza-associated hospitalizations and 64% of deaths during the 2015 to 2016 influenza season were in adults aged ≥65 years.[5] Although vaccination is the best way to protect against influenza and is recommended by the ACIP annually in older adults,[6] studies evaluating the efficacy of vaccination in this population have produced conflicting results.[7–9] A Cochrane review from 2010 concluded that available evidence to support the efficacy of influenza vaccination in adults aged ≥65 years was of poor quality.[10] A systematic review and meta-analysis from 2012 also concluded that evidence to assess the efficacy and effectiveness of influenza vaccination in adults aged 65 and older was inadequate.[9] A meta-analysis using test-negative design case-control studies from 2014 did find, however, that among community-dwelling older adults aged ≥60, the influenza vaccine was effective against laboratory-confirmed influenza during epidemic seasons when the vaccine was matched (odds ratio [OR] 0.69, 95% confidence interval [CI] 0.48–0.99). Additionally, vaccination was significantly effective during regional (match: OR 0.42, 95% CI 0.30–0.60; mismatch: OR 0.57, 95% CI 0.41–0.79) and widespread (match: 0.54, 95% CI 0.46–0.62; mismatch: OR 0.72, 95% CI 0.60–0.85) outbreaks.[11] A 2006 Cochrane review concluded that influenza vaccination was more effective in decreasing severity of disease, hospitalization, and mortality in adults aged ≥65 residing in long-term care compared with those living in the community.[12]

High-Dose Influenza Vaccination

Several studies have shown that adults aged ≥65 years respond less robustly to influenza vaccination (ie, produce fewer antibodies) compared with younger adults, likely a result of age-related immunosenescence.[13,14] To improve the efficacy of the influenza vaccine in older adults, a high-dose vaccine containing 4 times the amount of antigen (60 μg of hemagglutinin) compared with the standard-dose vaccine (15 μg of hemagglutinin) was developed and shown to stimulate more antibody production in this population.[13] The high-dose vaccine was approved by the Food and Drug Administration (FDA) in 2009 and was available for use in the 2010 to 2011 influenza season. A randomized controlled trial published in 2014 demonstrated that vaccination with the high-dose vaccine was 24.2% (95% CI 9.7–36.5) more effective in preventing laboratory-confirmed influenza in adults aged ≥65 years living in the United States compared with the standard-dose vaccination.[14] However, a subsequent large retrospective study in community-dwelling adults aged ≥65 in the United States did not find the high-dose vaccine to be more effective than the standard-dose vaccine for protecting against hospitalization for influenza or pneumonia (risk ratio 0.98; CI 0.68–1.40), except in a subgroup analysis of adults aged ≥85 years.[15] A more recent systematic review and meta-analysis that included 7 studies aimed to compare the efficacy and safety of the high-dose influenza vaccine with the standard-dose influenza vaccine in adults aged >65, found that adults receiving the high-dose vaccine had significantly less risk of developing laboratory-confirmed influenza infections (relative risk 0.76, 95% CI 0.65–0.90) compared with those receiving the standard-dose vaccine.[16]

The safety profile of the high-dose vaccine is similar to the standard-dose vaccine, although one study found that injection site pain (36% vs 24%) and fever $\geq 38°C$ (1.1% vs 0.3%) were higher in older adults receiving the high-dose vaccine.[13] The ACIP does not express a preference for either the high-dose or standard-dose influenza vaccination, as it is still unknown if the high-dose vaccine results in greater protection against influenza illness on a population level.[17] More studies regarding the efficacy and effectiveness of both the standard and high-dose influenza vaccinations and their cost-effectiveness are needed.

PNEUMOCOCCUS VACCINE

Pneumococcal disease causes a variety of infections in adults aged ≥ 65 years, including otitis media, pneumonia, meningitis, and sepsis, and is associated with significant morbidity and mortality in this age group.[18] The incidence of pneumococcal disease and pneumococcal pneumonia disproportionally affects adults aged ≥ 65 years, particularly in those with chronic medical comorbidities.[19] Pneumococcal cases account for more than 240,000 hospitalizations and approximately 16,000 deaths in older adults in the United States annually.[18] Pneumonia is the most common pneumococcal infection in older adults for which 80% of cases require hospitalization.[18] With the aging of the population, pneumococcal pneumonia hospitalizations are expected to increase to more than 750,000 by 2040, with an estimated cost of $2.5 billion annually.[20] There are currently 2 pneumococcal vaccines licensed for use in older adults in the United States, the 13-valent pneumococcal conjugate vaccine (PCV13) and the 23-valent pneumococcal polysaccharide vaccine (PPSV23).[21]

Pneumococcal Polysaccharide Vaccine

A vaccine against Streptococcus pneumonia was first developed in 1977 protecting against 14 types of pneumococcal bacteria, and then later expanded in 1983 to protect against 23 types of pneumococcal bacteria, known today as the 23-valent polysaccharide vaccine (PPSV23).[22] The ACIP currently recommends that adults aged ≥ 65 years receive PPSV23 at least once.[21] Additionally, ACIP recommends that adults who received PPSV23 before the age of 65 (recommended for other chronic medical conditions in younger adults) should receive another dose at age 65 or older if at least 5 years have passed since their previous dose.[21] These recommendations are based on few studies that have demonstrated efficacy of the PPSV23 against invasive pneumococcal diseases in older adults.[23,24] However, few studies evaluating the efficacy of the PPSV23 in older adults have revealed conflicting results, particularly in preventing pneumococcal pneumonia.[25] A 2013 systematic review and meta-analysis by Moberley and colleagues[24] assessed the efficacy of PPSV23 for preventing invasive pneumococcal disease, all-cause pneumonia, and all-cause mortality in adults. The investigators found that PPSV23 reduced the risk of invasive pneumococcal disease (OR 0.26, 95% CI 0.14–0.45) in the general adult population, including the subgroup of otherwise healthy individuals in high-income countries (OR 0.20, 95% CI 0.10–0.39), which included a large proportion of older adults. In this subgroup, however, there was no difference in all-cause pneumonia or mortality.[24] A more recent study published in 2017 sought to identify the serotype-specific effectiveness of the PPSV23 against pneumococcal pneumonia in adults 65 years and older. The investigators found that PPSV23 had low to moderate effectiveness against all pneumococcal pneumonia (27.4%) and against PPSV23-specific serotypes (33.5%).[26] Although not statistically significant, they found that protection was greater in adults aged <75 years.[26]

Pneumococcal Conjugate Vaccine

In September 2014, the ACIP released new recommendations that all adults aged ≥65 years receive the pneumococcal conjugate vaccine (PCV13), previously recommended only for use in younger children and those with high-risk medical conditions (eg, asplenia).[21] The rationale behind its use is that the conjugated protein vaccine might elicit a stronger immune response compared with the nonconjugated vaccine (PPSV23) in older adults.[27] The new guidelines are mostly based on results from a large randomized controlled trial published in 2015, concluding that among adults aged ≥65 years, PCV13 was found to be effective in preventing (1) vaccine-type community-acquired pneumonia (vaccine efficacy 45.6%, 95% CI 21.8%–62.5%), (2) confirmed nonbacteremic and noninvasive community-acquired pneumonia (vaccine efficacy 45%, 95% CI 14.2%–65.3%), and (3) invasive pneumococcal disease (vaccine efficacy 75%, CI 41.4%–90,8%).[28] There was no difference in all-cause mortality. However, this study was done in older adults living in the Netherlands who had not received the PPSV23. As opposed to the United States, the PPSV23 was not routinely administered to adults aged ≥65 years in the Netherlands during the trial period. Thus, the efficacy of PCV13 to older adults already vaccinated with PPSV23 is unknown. Additionally, widespread vaccination of younger children with PCV13 has likely reduced the burden of pneumococcal disease in older adults through herd immunity.[29] Although currently recommended in the United States, many developed countries do not recommend the routine use of PCV13 in adults aged ≥65 without high-risk comorbidities.[30] See **Fig. 1** for the recommended pneumococcal vaccination schedule in older adults.

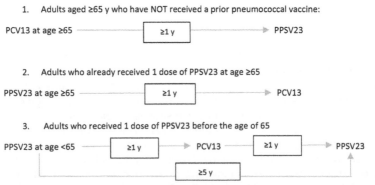

Fig. 1. Recommended pneumococcal vaccination schedule in adults aged ≥65. (*Adapted from* Kobayashi M, Bennett NM, Gierke R, et al. Intervals between PCV13 and PPSV23 vaccines: recommendations of the Advisory Committee on Immunization Practices (ACIP). MMWR Morb Mortal Wkly Rep 2015;64(34):944–7.)

VARICELLA-ZOSTER VIRUS VACCINE

Older adults are at increased risk of varicella virus reactivation (ie, herpes zoster or shingles) and for greater disease severity because of age-associated changes in cell-mediated immunity.[31,32] Herpes zoster vaccination has been shown to decrease the risk of developing herpes zoster and postherpetic neuralgia by boosting cell-mediated immunity to the varicella virus.[32–34] There are 2 varicella-zoster vaccines approved for use in older adults, the live attenuated zoster vaccine and the inactived subunit herpes zoster vaccine.[34,35]

Inactivated Subunit Herpes Zoster Vaccine

The inactivated subunit herpes zoster vaccine contains recombinant varicella-zoster virus glycoprotein E in combination with an adjuvant (ASO1B). It was found to significantly reduce the risks of herpes zoster and post-herpetic neuralgia in adults aged ≥70 years old who were followed for a mean of 3.7 years. In this study, 23 participants who received the new vaccine developed herpes zoster compared with 223 of those receiving placebo, resulting in a vaccine efficacy of 89.9% (95% CI, 84.2–93.7). The vaccine efficacy for prevention of post-herpetic neuralgia was 88.8% (CI, 68.7–97.1).[34] The ACIP now recommends the inactivated herpes zoster subunit vaccine for:

- Prevention of herpes zoster and related complications for immunocompetent adults aged ≥50 years.
- Prevention of herpes zoster and related complications for immunocompetent adults who previously received the live attenuated herpes zoster vaccine.
- Preferred over the live attenuated herpes zoster vaccine for prevention of herpes zoster and related complications.

Although the ACIP issued these new recommendations, endorsement from the director of the CDC is still pending, and recommendations for use in immunocompromised older adults and those with a history of herpes zoster have not been released.

Live Attenuated Herpes Zoster Vaccine

The live attenuated herpes zoster vaccine is approved in adults aged ≥ 60 years old. A randomized placebo-controlled trial comparing the efficacy of herpes zoster vaccination with placebo in adults aged ≥60 described the following results[36]:

- Efficacy of herpes zoster vaccine in prevention of zoster was 51.3% over 3 years compared with placebo (1.6% vs 3.3%, $P<.001$).
- Mean duration of pain and discomfort was shorter in the vaccinated group compared with placebo (21 days vs 24 days, $P = .03$).
- Efficacy for prevention of postherpetic neuralgia was overall 66.5% (0.46 cases vs 1.38 cases per 1000 person-years).

A retrospective cohort study in 2011 in community-dwelling adults aged ≥60 years living in the United States also found that the incidence of herpes zoster was lower in vaccinated adults (hazard ratio 0.45; 95% CI 0.42–0.48) compared with unvaccinated adults. The number of herpes zoster cases among vaccinated individuals was 6.4 per 1000 person-years compared with 13.0 per 1000 person-years in unvaccinated adults. The vaccine was associated with lower incidence among all age groups, including those aged ≥70.[37] A systematic review and meta-analysis published in 2016 also concluded that herpes zoster vaccine was effective in preventing cases of herpes zoster, although noted that protection beyond 3 years was uncertain.[38] The Shingles Prevention Study, which followed adults aged ≥60 who received the herpes zoster vaccine, concluded that the clinical efficacy of zoster vaccination was limited beyond 5 years after vaccination.[39]

Herpes Zoster Vaccine Administration

ACIP now prefers that all adults aged $\geq$50 years be vaccinated with the inactivated subunit vaccine. This vaccine is given in 2 doses, approximately 2 months.[34] However, final schedule recommendations and clarifications for those with a prior history of herpes zoster are still pending. The live attenuated herpes zoster vaccine is approved for adults aged $\geq$60 years, regardless of whether they have had a prior episode of herpes zoster.[35,40] For patients with a known history of herpes zoster (ie, shingles), administration of the herpes zoster vaccine should be delayed at least a year to provide optimal immune response.[40] Vaccination should be given to all adults even if history of primary varicella virus infection (ie, chicken pox) is unknown, and there is no need to perform serologic testing to determine varicella immunity.[35,41] ACIP considers that adults born in the United States before 1980 are immune to varicella. If serologic evidence demonstrating that adults are not immune to varicella becomes available, older adults should be offered varicella vaccine and not the zoster vaccine. The live attenuated herpes zoster vaccine can be given to older adults with comorbidities; however, because it contains live virus, should be avoided in patients with moderate to severe immunosuppression due to theoretic risk of potential disseminated herpes zoster infection.[35,41] The inactivated subunit herpes zoster vaccine is recommended in immunocompetent adults and has not yet been approved or recommended for those with moderate to severe immunosuppression.

TETANUS, DIPHTHERIA, PERTUSSIS VACCINATION
Tetanus and Diphtheria

Tetanus and diphtheria are now rare diseases in the United States, although the incidence of both tetanus and diphtheria are highest in older adults.[42] Tetanus is an infection caused by *Clostridium tetani* and because the most common cause of infection is unpredictable acute injuries, vaccination remains the best way to prevent infection.[42] Although the tetanus vaccine has been available and recommended since 1940 in the United States, data show that fewer than 30% of adults aged $\geq$70 in the United States have protective levels of tetanus antibody.[43] The CDC estimates that only 40% to 60% of adults aged $\geq$65 received any form of the tetanus vaccine within the past 10 years.[4,44] Similar to tetanus, a cross-sectional survey found that only 30% of adults aged $\geq$60 living in the United States had protective levels of diphtheria antibody, likely a result of low vaccination rates.[45]

Pertussis

Pertussis is an acute, infectious cough illness that remains endemic in the United States despite longstanding routine childhood vaccination.[46] Immunity to pertussis wanes approximately 5 to 10 years after completion of childhood vaccination, leaving adolescents and adults susceptible to pertussis. The National Disease Surveillance System reported that among adults aged $\geq$65 years old there have been an average 318 cases of documented pertussis in the United States annually from 2000 to 2012 (range of 71–719 cases per year). Because older adults often present with pertussis atypically, the burden of disease actually may be higher.[46]

Recommended Vaccination Schedule

Although previously recommended only to adults aged $\geq$65 years old if in close contact with infants, the FDA approved the tetanus diphtheria acellular pertussis vaccine

(Tdap) for use in older adults in 2011 and the ACIP began recommending the Tdap vaccination for all adults ≥65 years old in 2012.[46]

HEPATITIS VACCINATIONS

There are 2 vaccinations against hepatitis infections available for older adults: hepatitis A vaccine and hepatitis B vaccine. Recommendations for hepatitis vaccination in older adults are similar to younger adults, and are guided by specific risk factors and not age alone.[6] As many older adults are living longer, healthier lives, it is important for clinicians to ask about risk factors, including sexual activity and travel history.

Hepatitis A

ACIP recommends hepatitis A vaccination in the following situations:

1. Travel outside of the United States
2. Men who have sex with men
3. Illicit drug users (both injection and noninjection)
4. Individuals with chronic liver disease (especially those with chronic hepatitis B and/or hepatitis C infection)
5. Individuals with clotting factor disorders

Hepatitis B

ACIP recommends consideration of hepatitis B vaccination in the following situations:

1. Multiple sexual partners
2. History of a sexually transmitted disease
3. Men who have sex with men
4. Illicit drug users (both injection and noninjection)
5. Living with someone who has chronic hepatitis B
6. On hemodialysis
7. Travel to countries with moderate to high rates of hepatitis B
8. Exposure to blood at work

See **Table 1** for the recommended vaccination schedule for vaccines discussed previously.

BARRIERS TO VACCINATION IN OLDER ADULTS
Cost of Vaccinations

Most vaccinations are covered by Medicare. More than 90% of Medicare beneficiaries have Medicare Part B, which covers seasonal influenza vaccinations, pneumococcal vaccinations, and hepatitis B vaccinations. Other vaccinations, including herpes zoster and Tdap, are covered by Medicare Part D and are subject to deductibles and copays for each vaccine.[47] Approximately 71% of older adults are enrolled in Medicare Part D. Although routine vaccinations are covered by Medicare, cost has been found to be a significant barrier to vaccine administration in older adults.[48] This is particularly true for the herpes zoster vaccine, for which only 20% to 30% of older adults actually receive.[4] In a study by Hurley and colleagues[49] in 2010, assessing barriers to herpes zoster vaccination in primary care, the most frequently reported barrier to vaccination was financial. Only 45% of primary care physicians (PCPs) were aware that the herpes zoster vaccine was reimbursed through Medicare Part D. Additionally, 12% of PCPs reported

Table 1
Recommended vaccination schedule of selected vaccines in older adults as recommended by the Centers for Disease Control and Prevention Advisory Committee on Immunization Practices

Vaccine	Recommended Dose/Schedule
Flu (*Influenza*)	High-dose or standard inactivated influenza vaccine yearly
Pneumococcal conjugated (PCV13)	One dose before receiving PPSV23 in adults aged ≥65 y or ≥1 y after adults aged ≥65 y receiving PPSV23[a]
Pneumococcal polysaccharide (PPSV23)	One dose in adults aged ≥65 or 5 y after previous dose if given before age 65
Shingles (*Zoster*)	Two doses of the inactivated subunit vaccine in immunocompetent adults ≥50 years old is preferred over the live zoster vaccine[b]
Hepatitis A	Two doses based on risk factors[c]
Hepatitis B	Three doses based on risk factors[d]
Td (*Tetanus, diphtheria*)/Tdap (*Tetanus, diphtheria, pertussis*)	Tdap once with Td booster every 10 y

For complete list visit: https://www.cdc.gov/vaccines/schedules/downloads/adult/adult-combined-schedule.pdf.

Abbreviation: Tdap, tetanus diphtheria acellular pertussis vaccine.

[a] See **Fig. 1** for dosing schedule if already received PPSV23.

[b] Adults who have already received the live attenuated zoster vaccine should also receive the inactivated subunit vaccine. Excludes patients with severe acquired or primary immunodeficiency. Although this recommendation was endorsed by the ACIP, formal endorsement from the director of the CDC is still pending.

[c] Risk factors include men who have sex with men, persons who use illicit drugs, persons with chronic liver disease or who receive clotting factor concentrates, or international travelers.

[d] Risk factors include sexually active persons not in a monogamous relationship, injection drug users, men who have sex with men, those being evaluated for a sexually transmitted infection, diabetic patients, those potentially exposed to blood or body fluids (eg, health care workers), persons with end-stage renal disease (including those on hemodialysis), human immunodeficiency virus infection, persons with chronic liver disease, household contacts and sex partners of hepatitis B–positive persons, international travelers, all adults in institutions and nonresidential daycare facilities, or persons with developmental disabilities.

that they stopped administering herpes zoster vaccine in their office because of cost and reimbursement issues.

Another study by Hurley and colleagues[50] in 2017, exploring financial barriers to PCPs recommending vaccinations to their adult patients, found that a significant proportion of PCPs did not recommend vaccines because they thought that (1) a patient's insurance would not cover it (35%) or (2) the patient could be vaccinated more affordably elsewhere (38%). PCPs also reported that patients were less likely to decline vaccines for which no copay was required (eg, vaccines covered by Medicare Part B) and more likely to refuse vaccines covered by Medicare Part D (eg, herpes zoster and Tdap) because of the additional copay.[48,49] There were also concerns from PCPs about inadequate reimbursement for vaccinations, which influenced their willingness to recommend them.[48]

Similar financial issues were a known barrier to pediatric immunizations in the United States. The development of Vaccines for Children (VFC), a program designed to ensure that cost did not prohibit children from receiving vaccinations, has been successful in improving and sustaining a high vaccination rate in this population.[51] A similar program specifically for older adults also may be beneficial in increasing the vaccination rate; however, no such program has yet been developed.

Racial and Ethnic Barriers

There continues to be significant racial/ethnic gaps in coverage for all vaccinations recommended for older adults, with white individuals having the highest vaccination rates. For the pneumococcal vaccine, coverage among white individuals aged ≥65 was approximately 65%, compared with black individuals at approximately 50%, Hispanic individuals 45%, and Asian individuals 48%.[4] In a cross-sectional survey of patients with Medicare in the United States, white patients had significantly higher odds of vaccination than did black patients (OR 1.52, 95% CI 1.35–1.71), after adjusting for patient, physician, health system, and area-level characteristics.[52] Further studies and programs addressing racial and ethnic barriers to vaccinations are needed.

Misconceptions

Other common barriers to vaccinations in older adults are associated with misconceptions about vaccinations and include (1) beliefs that vaccines cause illness, (2) beliefs that vaccines are generally ineffective, and (3) belief that older adults are at little risk for vaccine-preventable illnesses.[53] In 2011, the National Vaccine Advisory Committee developed a guidance document with a summary of recommendations to address barriers to vaccination in adults.[1] It is important to highlight that health care professionals can significantly influence vaccination rates. Several studies have found that physician counseling and recommendations significantly improve vaccination uptake in older adults.[50,53] **Fig. 2** reviews the percentage of older adults receiving appropriate vaccinations compared with all adults for which each vaccine is recommended.

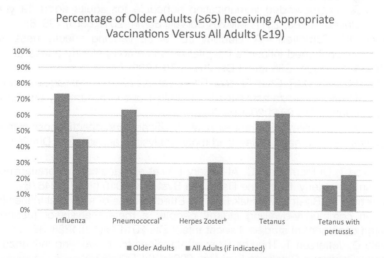

Fig. 2. Vaccination coverage in older adults. [a] Pneumococcal vaccine is indicated in adults younger than 65 years at increased risk. [b] Herpes zoster rates are compared in this chart between adults ≥65 years and ≥60 years. (*Data from* Williams WW, Lu PJ, O'Halloran A, et al. Surveillance of vaccination coverage among adult populations—United States, 2015. MMWR Surveill Summ 2017;66(11):1–28.)

SUMMARY

Vaccines are crucial to improving the health of older adults. Although older adults have a blunted immune response to vaccines, they remain one of the most important prevention strategies for several devastating illnesses that most commonly affect this population. Despite national campaigns highlighting the benefits of vaccinations, overall vaccination rates in this age group remain low, especially among minorities.[4] Clinician recommendations largely influence whether or not patients receive vaccinations and are an important target for improving vaccination coverage. Further studies exploring costs and other barriers to vaccination specifically in older adults are needed.

REFERENCES

1. National Vaccine Advisory Committee. A pathway to leadership for adult immunization: recommendations of the National Vaccine Advisory Committee: approved by the National Vaccine Advisory Committee on June 14, 2011. Public Health Rep 2012;127(Suppl 1):1–42.
2. Healthy people 2020. Available at: https://www.healthypeople.gov/2020/topics-objectives/topic/immunization-and-infectious-diseases. Accessed May 17, 2017.
3. Castle SC, Uyemura K, Fulop T, et al. Host resistance and immune responses in advanced age. Clin Geriatr Med 2007;23(3):463–79, v.
4. Williams WW, Lu PJ, O'Halloran A, et al. Surveillance of vaccination coverage among adult populations—United States, 2015. MMWR Surveill Summ 2017; 66(11):1–28.
5. Rolfes MA, Foppa IM, Garg S, et al. Estimated influenza illnesses, medical visits, hospitalizations, and deaths averted by vaccination in the United States. 2016; Available at: https://www.cdc.gov/flu/about/disease/2015-16.htm. Accessed May 17, 2017.
6. Kim DK, Riley LE, Harriman KH, et al. Advisory Committee on Immunization Practices recommended immunization schedule for adults aged 19 years or older—United States, 2017. MMWR Surveill Summ 2017;66(5):136–8.
7. Kwong JC, Campitelli MA, Gubbay JB, et al. Vaccine effectiveness against laboratory-confirmed influenza hospitalizations among elderly adults during the 2010-2011 season. Clin Infect Dis 2013;57(6):820–7.
8. Talbot HK, Griffin MR, Chen Q, et al. Effectiveness of seasonal vaccine in preventing confirmed influenza-associated hospitalizations in community dwelling older adults. J Infect Dis 2011;203(4):500–8.
9. Osterholm MT, Kelley NS, Sommer A, et al. Efficacy and effectiveness of influenza vaccines: a systematic review and meta-analysis. Lancet Infect Dis 2012;12(1): 36–44.
10. Jefferson T, Di Pietrantonj C, Al-Ansary LA, et al. Vaccines for preventing influenza in the elderly. Cochrane Database Syst Rev 2010;(2):CD004876.
11. Darvishian M, Bijlsma MJ, Hak E, et al. Effectiveness of seasonal influenza vaccine in community-dwelling elderly people: a meta-analysis of test-negative design case-control studies. Lancet Infect Dis 2014;14(12):1228–39.
12. Rivetti D, Jefferson T, Thomas R, et al. Vaccines for preventing influenza in the elderly. Cochrane Database Syst Rev 2006;(3):CD004876.
13. Falsey AR, Treanor JJ, Tornieporth N, et al. Randomized, double-blind controlled phase 3 trial comparing the immunogenicity of high-dose and standard-dose influenza vaccine in adults 65 years of age and older. J Infect Dis 2009;200(2): 172–80.

14. DiazGranados CA, Dunning AJ, Kimmel M, et al. Efficacy of high-dose versus standard-dose influenza vaccine in older adults. New Engl J Med 2014;371(7): 635–45.

15. Richardson DM, Medvedeva EL, Roberts CB, et al, Centers for Disease Control and Prevention Epicenter Program. Comparative effectiveness of high-dose versus standard-dose influenza vaccination in community-dwelling veterans. Clin Infect Dis 2015;61(2):171–6.

16. Wilkinson K, Wei Y, Szwajcer A, et al. Efficacy and safety of high-dose influenza vaccine in elderly adults: a systematic review and meta-analysis. Vaccine 2017; 35(21):2775–80.

17. Centers for Disease Control and Prevention (CDC). Licensure of a high-dose inactivated influenza vaccine for persons aged >or=65 years (Fluzone High-Dose) and guidance for use—United States, 2010. MMWR Morb Mortal Wkly Rep 2010; 59(16):485–6.

18. Huang SS, Johnson KM, Ray GT, et al. Healthcare utilization and cost of pneumococcal disease in the United States. Vaccine 2011;29(18):3398–412.

19. Wagenvoort GH, Knol MJ, de Melker HE, et al. Risk and outcomes of invasive pneumococcal disease in adults with underlying conditions in the post-PCV7 era, The Netherlands. Vaccine 2016;34(3):334–40.

20. Wroe PC, Finkelstein JA, Ray GT, et al. Aging population and future burden of pneumococcal pneumonia in the United States. J Infect Dis 2012;205(10): 1589–92.

21. Tomczyk S, Bennett NM, Stoecker C, et al. Use of 13-valent pneumococcal conjugate vaccine and 23-valent pneumococcal polysaccharide vaccine among adults aged >/=65 years: recommendations of the Advisory Committee on Immunization Practices (ACIP). MMWR Morb Mortal Wkly Rep 2014;63(37):822–5.

22. Centers for Disease Control and Prevention. In: Hamborsky JKA, Wolfe S, editors. Epidemology and prevention of vaccine-preventable diseases. 13th edition. Washington, DC: Public Health Foundation; 2015.

23. Jackson LA, Neuzil KM, Yu O, et al. Effectiveness of pneumococcal polysaccharide vaccine in older adults. New Engl J Med 2003;348(18):1747–55.

24. Moberley S, Holden J, Tatham DP, et al. Vaccines for preventing pneumococcal infection in adults. Cochrane Database Syst Rev 2013;(1):CD000422.

25. Huss A, Scott P, Stuck AE, et al. Efficacy of pneumococcal vaccination in adults: a meta-analysis. CMAJ 2009;180(1):48–58.

26. Suzuki M, Dhoubhadel BG, Ishifuji T, et al. Serotype-specific effectiveness of 23-valent pneumococcal polysaccharide vaccine against pneumococcal pneumonia in adults aged 65 years or older: a multicentre, prospective, test-negative design study. Lancet Infect Dis 2017;17(3):313–21.

27. French N, Gordon SB, Mwalukomo T, et al. A trial of a 7-valent pneumococcal conjugate vaccine in HIV-infected adults. N Engl J Med 2010;362(9):812–22.

28. Bonten MJ, Huijts SM, Bolkenbaas M, et al. Polysaccharide conjugate vaccine against pneumococcal pneumonia in adults. N Engl J Med 2015;372(12): 1114–25.

29. Centers for Disease Control and Prevention. Epidemiology and prevention of vaccine-preventable diseases. In: Hamborsky JKA, Wolfe S, editors. Use of 13-valent pneumococcal conjugate vaccine and 23-valent pneumococcal polysaccharide vaccine among adults aged ≥ 65 years: recommendations of the Advisory Committee on Immunization Practices (ACIP). 13th edition. Washington, DC: Public Health Foundation; 2015. p. 279–94.

30. NHS. Pneumococcal vaccine. 2016. Available at: http://www.nhs.uk/Conditions/vaccinations/Pages/pneumococcal-vaccination.aspx. Accessed October 5, 2017.

31. Levin MJ, Smith JG, Kaufhold RM, et al. Decline in varicella-zoster virus (VZV)-specific cell-mediated immunity with increasing age and boosting with a high-dose VZV vaccine. J Infect Dis 2003;188(9):1336–44.

32. Weinberg A, Zhang JH, Oxman MN, et al. Varicella-zoster virus-specific immune responses to herpes zoster in elderly participants in a trial of a clinically effective zoster vaccine. J Infect Dis 2009;200(7):1068–77.

33. Levin MJ, Oxman MN, Zhang JH, et al. Varicella-zoster virus-specific immune responses in elderly recipients of a herpes zoster vaccine. J Infect Dis 2008;197(6):825–35.

34. Cunningham AL, Lal H, Kovac M, et al. Efficacy of the herpes zoster subunit vaccine in adults 70 years of age or older. New Engl J Med 2016;375(11):1019–32.

35. Hales CM, Harpaz R, Ortega-Sanchez I, et al, Centers for Disease Control and Prevention (CDC). Update on recommendations for use of herpes zoster vaccine. MMWR Morb Mortal Wkly Rep 2014;63(33):729–31.

36. Oxman MN, Levin MJ, Johnson GR, et al. A vaccine to prevent herpes zoster and postherpetic neuralgia in older adults. New Engl J Med 2005;352(22):2271–84.

37. Tseng HF, Smith N, Harpaz R, et al. Herpes zoster vaccine in older adults and the risk of subsequent herpes zoster disease. JAMA 2011;305(2):160–6.

38. Gagliardi AM, Andriolo BN, Torloni MR, et al. Vaccines for preventing herpes zoster in older adults. Cochrane Database Syst Rev 2016;(3):CD008858.

39. Morrison VA, Johnson GR, Schmader KE, et al. Long-term persistence of zoster vaccine efficacy. Clin Infect Dis 2015;60(6):900–9.

40. Morrison VA, Oxman MN, Levin MJ, et al. Safety of zoster vaccine in elderly adults following documented herpes zoster. J Infect Dis 2013;208(4):559–63.

41. Harpaz R, Ortega-Sanchez IR, Seward JF, Advisory Committee On Immunization Practices Centers for Disease Control and Prevention. Prevention of herpes zoster: recommendations of the Advisory Committee on Immunization Practices (ACIP). MMWR Recommendations Rep 2008;57(RR-5):1–30 [quiz: CE32-34].

42. Centers for Disease Control and Prevention (CDC). Tetanus surveillance—United States, 2001-2008. MMWR Morb Mortal Wkly Rep 2011;60(12):365–9.

43. Gergen PJ, McQuillan GM, Kiely M, et al. A population-based serologic survey of immunity to tetanus in the United States. New Engl J Med 1995;332(12):761–6.

44. Singleton JA, Greby SM, Wooten KG, et al. Influenza, pneumococcal, and tetanus toxoid vaccination of adults–United States, 1993-7. MMWR CDC Surveill Summ 2000;49(9):39–62.

45. McQuillan GM, Kruszon-Moran D, Deforest A, et al. Serologic immunity to diphtheria and tetanus in the United States. Ann Intern Med 2002;136(9):660–6.

46. Kretsinger K, Broder KR, Cortese MM, et al. Preventing tetanus, diphtheria, and pertussis among adults: use of tetanus toxoid, reduced diphtheria toxoid and acellular pertussis vaccine recommendations of the Advisory Committee on Immunization Practices (ACIP) and recommendation of ACIP, supported by the Healthcare Infection Control Practices Advisory Committee (HICPAC), for use of Tdap among health-care personnel. MMWR Recommendations Rep 2006;55(RR-17):1–37.

47. Aging NCo. Vaccines: what Medicare pays for. 2016; Available at: https://www.ncoa.org/wp-content/uploads/medicare-vaccines.pdf. Accessed May 23, 2017.

48. Hurley LP, Bridges CB, Harpaz R, et al. U.S. physicians' perspective of adult vaccine delivery. Ann Intern Med 2014;160(3):161.

49. Hurley LP, Lindley MC, Harpaz R, et al. Barriers to the use of herpes zoster vaccine. Ann Intern Med 2010;152(9):555–60.
50. Hurley LP, Lindley MC, Allison MA, et al. Primary care physicians' perspective on financial issues and adult immunization in the era of the Affordable Care Act. Vaccine 2017;35(4):647–54.
51. Whitney CG, Zhou F, Singleton J, et al. Benefits from immunization during the vaccines for children program era—United States, 1994-2013. MMWR Morbidity Mortality Weekly Rep 2014;63(16):352–5.
52. O'Malley AS, Forrest CB. Immunization disparities in older Americans: determinants and future research needs. Am J Prev Med 2006;31(2):150–8.
53. Nagata JM, Hernandez-Ramos I, Kurup AS, et al. Social determinants of health and seasonal influenza vaccination in adults >/=65 years: a systematic review of qualitative and quantitative data. BMC Public Health 2013;13:388.

Exercise and Older Adults

Jorge Camilo Mora, MD, MPH[a],*, Willy M. Valencia, MD[b]

KEYWORDS

- Geriatrics • Preventive medicine • Exercise • Primary care • Risk reduction behavior

KEY POINTS

- Regular physical activity is essential for healthy aging and offers a range of health benefits, including reduced risk of all-cause mortality, chronic disease, and premature death.
- Because physical inactivity is prevalent, greater focus needs to be placed on integrating exercise into care plans and counseling, and developing community partnerships supporting exercise opportunities.
- Older adults should be as physically active as their abilities and conditions allow. For substantial health benefits, older adults need at least 150 minutes of aerobic exercise weekly.
- Physical activity planning and counseling for patients needs to take account of the impact of prescribed medications, nutrition, injuries, hip and knee arthroplasties, and chronic conditions.

INTRODUCTION

Regular physical activity is essential for healthy aging and supports positive mental health. It can help to delay, prevent, or manage many costly and challenging chronic diseases faced by older adults. It can also reduce the risk of moderate or severe functional limitations in older adults and the risk of premature death.[1–3]

Physical Inactivity Among Older Adults

Prevalence of physical inactivity

Despite clear benefits of physical activity, 27.5% of US adults 50 and over, approximately 31 million persons, self-reported as inactive.[1,4] Inactivity is defined by the US Department of Health and Human Services as participating in no activity beyond baseline activities of daily living.[1] The prevalence of inactivity increases with advancement in age: adults aged 50 to 64 years (25.4%), 65 to 74 years (26.9%), and 75 years and older (35.3%).[4]

Disclosure Statement: The authors have nothing to disclose.
[a] FIU Herbert Wertheim College of Medicine, 11200 Southwest 8th Street, AHC4 456A, Miami, FL 33199, USA; [b] Department of Public Health Sciences, Miami VA Healthcare System, Geriatrics Research, Education & Clinical Center (GRECC), University of Miami Miller School of Medicine, 1201 Northwest 16th Street, 11 GRC, Miami, FL 33125, USA
* Corresponding author.
E-mail address: jcmora@fiu.edu

Clin Geriatr Med 34 (2018) 145–162
https://doi.org/10.1016/j.cger.2017.08.007
0749-0690/18/© 2017 Elsevier Inc. All rights reserved.
geriatric.theclinics.com

Chronic disease and physical inactivity
Among adults with at least 1 of 7 chronic diseases, the prevalence of inactivity was higher (31.9%) than among those not reporting any (19.2%).[1,4] The pervasiveness of inactivity ranges depending on the chronic disease: arthritis (33%), cancer (31.6%), coronary heart disease (37.2%), chronic obstructive pulmonary disease (44.4%), depressive disorder (38%), diabetes (38%), stroke (43%).[4]

Effects of physical inactivity
There are multiple epidemiologic studies showing a reduction of all-cause mortality, disability, and cardiovascular disease in older adults who exercise regularly. Adherence to physical activity that burns more than 1000 kcal/week is associated with up to 30% reduction in all case mortality. Further benefits are achieved with higher energy expenditures.[5]

Interventions to Increase Physical Activity Among Older Adults

The role of primary care
Primary care practice provides a powerful opportunity for exercise counseling and prescription. However, few physicians routinely gather an exercise history or provide explicit exercise instructions to patients. In a national survey, insufficient time and inadequate knowledge and/or experience were identified as the 2 major barriers to exercise counseling.[6] A third barrier is reimbursement structures, such as Medicare and Medicaid Services, which do not include exercise counseling for nonobese older adults. One strategy for overcoming these barriers is for primary care practices to form partnerships with senior centers, YMCAs, and local departments of aging to ensure that their patients receive support and opportunities to improve physical activity.[1–3,7,8]

Social determinants of health and physical activity
Substantial literature has established that the conditions in the social and physical environments in which people are born, live, work, and age bear an important role in determining health outcomes across the life stages.[9] Studies highlight the negative health implications of structural barriers to increasing physical activity among older adults.[1,4] One national study shows that physical activity resources—such as gyms, parks, fitness clubs, and walking/bike trails—are inequitably distributed among different demographic and socioeconomic populations.[10] These findings among others support recent calls for cross-sector, collaborative solutions to support physical activity among older adults.[1,3,11]

CURRENT EXERCISE RECOMMENDATIONS FOR OLDER ADULTS
Physical Activity Guidelines

Excepting cases where contraindicated, physical activity should be part of every older adult's plan of care.[12] Older adults who participate in any amount of exercise gain some health benefits. The level of effort for physical activity should be relative to the older adult's level of fitness and ability.[3]

Key Recommendations for Exercise Beyond Regular Amount of Daily Activities

According to US Department of Health and Human Services' *2008 Physical Guidelines for Americans*[3] and others,[13,14] older adults should aim to achieve weekly exercise goals beyond routine activities in daily living to attain health benefits **(Table 1).**

Table 1
Regular exercise guidelines for older adults

Exercise Type	Recommendation	Examples
Aerobic and endurance activities	• Any modality of aerobic or endurance activity that does not impose excessive orthopedic stress. • Older adults should do at least 150 min a week of moderate intensity (5 or 6),[a] or 75 min a week of vigorous intensity (7 or 8)[a] aerobic physical activity for substantial health benefits. • Older adults may incrementally build up stamina, but should aim to perform these activities in episodes of at least 10 min, and preferably spread across 3 or more days. • Additional and more extensive health benefits are gained by extending this regimen to 300 min a week of moderate intensity (5 or 6),[a] or 150 min a week of vigorous intensity (7 or 8)[a] aerobic physical activity.	Walking, dancing, swimming, water aerobics, jogging, aerobic exercise classes, bicycle riding (stationary or on a path), some activities of gardening, such as raking and pushing a lawn mower, tennis, golf (without a cart).
Muscle-strengthening activities	• Progressive weight training program, weight bearing, or weight bearing calisthenics. • No specific amount of time is recommended for muscle strengthening, but muscle-strengthening exercises should be performed to the point at which it would be difficult to do another repetition without help. When resistance training is used to enhance muscle strength, 1 set of 8 to 12 repetitions of each exercise is effective, although 2 or 3 sets may be more effective. • At least 2 times per week, with moderate to vigorous intensity ($\geq$6).[a] • Development of muscle strength and endurance is progressive over time. This means that gradual increases in the amount of weight or the days per week of exercise will result in stronger muscles.	Exercises using exercise bands, weight machines, hand-held weights, callisthenic exercises (body weight provides resistance to movement), digging, lifting, and carrying as part of gardening, carrying groceries, some yoga exercises, some tai chi exercises.

(*continued on next page*)

Table 1
(continued)

Exercise Type	Recommendation	Examples
Flexibility	• Any activities that maintain or increase flexibility using sustained stretches for each major muscle group. • Minimum of 2 times per week. • This type of exercise is recommended to maintain the normal range of motion for daily activities, and is typically joined with warm-up or cool-down surrounding aerobic or muscle-strengthening activities.	Neck stretch, shoulder stretch, shoulder and upper arm raise, upper body stretch, chest stretch, back stretch, ankle stretch, back of leg stretch, thigh stretch, hip stretch, lower back, calf stretch.[b]
Balance activities for older adults at risk of falls and/or with mobility problems	• Reduction in falls is seen for participants in programs that include balance and moderate-intensity[a] muscle-strengthening activities for 90 min a week plus moderate intensity[a] walking for about 1 h a week. • Older adults at risk of falls should do balance training 3 or more days a week and do standardized exercises from a program demonstrated to reduce falls. • Progressively difficult postures that gradually reduce the base of support, dynamic movements that perturb the center of gravity, and stressing postural muscle groups. • In older adults at increased risk of falls, strong evidence shows that regular physical activity is safe and reduces the risk of falls.	Backward walking, sideways walking, heel walking, toe walking, and standing from a sitting position. The exercises can increase in difficulty by progressing from holding onto a stable support (like furniture) while doing the exercises to doing them without support. Tai chi exercises also may help to prevent falls.

[a] On a scale of 0 to 10, where 0 is the level of effort of sitting and 10 is maximal effort, the level of self-perceived effort distinguishes between moderate intensity activity (5 or 6) and vigorous intensity activity (7 or 8).
[b] List of flexibility exercises taken retrieved from US Department of Health & Human Services, National Institute of Health, NIH SeniorHealth. Flexibility Exercises. 2010. Available at: https://nihseniorhealth.gov/exerciseandphysicalactivityexercisestotry/flexibilityexercises/01.html. Accessed June 3, 2017.
Data from 2008 Physical Activity Guidelines for Americans. Washington, DC: U.S. Department of Health and Human Services; 2008. ODPHP Publication No. U0036.

EXERCISE AND MEDICATIONS

Prescription drug usage is prevalent among older adults.[15] People 65 years of age and older comprise 12% of the US population but account for 34% of prescription medication use and 30% of over-the-counter medication use.[16] Based on US survey data, more than 90% of people in this group took at least 1 prescription medication in the prior 30 days, and 39% take 5 or more medications on a regular basis.[15] Some of the most commonly prescribed medications can negatively impair exercise performance (**Table 2**).

EXERCISE AND NUTRITION IN OLDER ADULTS

Nutritional assessment and support predominately focuses on older adults with frailty. However, 8.3% of adults 65 and older live in households with food insecurity.[30] The prevalence increases to 9.2% among the elderly who live alone.[30] The overall energy needs during exercise declines with age because of decrease in lean body mass and resting metabolic rate. Nevertheless, exercise increases both calorie and micronutrient needs. Exercise increases metabolic pathways that use thiamine (vitamin B_1), riboflavin (vitamin B_2), and pyridoxine (vitamin B_6).[31] It is important that nutritional counseling accompany physical activity planning.[32]

Dehydration

Older adults are also more susceptible to dehydration because of a decreased perception of thirst, decreased renal function, and slower response to rehydration. These factors can lead to inadequate hydration during exercise. Older adults should be made aware of the risk of dehydration and advise how to safely avoid this.[33]

EXERCISE AND INJURIES IN OLDER ADULTS

With aging, ligaments and tendons experience decreased compliance and vascularity. Skeletal muscles show decreasing mitochondrial volume, increased collagen content, and decreased flexibility. Meniscus and articular cartilage lose the ability to dissipate stress and develop chondromalacia (cumulative damage).[34] With an annual rate of injuries related to regular exercise at around 20%,[35] injuries are frequently related to repetitive stress and overuse,[36] and commonly occur in the lower extremities.[35] Among the most common is muscle strain,[37] precipitated by a decreased capacity to absorb energy in aging muscles. Tendinosis is also common, because microtrauma and lack of vascularity make tendons stiffer and more prone to inflammation. Because healing takes longer in older adults, they are especially vulnerable to injuries in endurance sports.[37] These studies accentuate the importance of musculoskeletal screening and gradual progression.

EXERCISE AFTER HIP AND KNEE ARTHROPLASTY

Some of the main goals with any arthroplasty are to improve the patient's quality of life, and reduce pain and disability. In addition, it is expected that patients have higher mobility and better endurance. Although higher activity is associated with greater postoperative satisfaction, it can also increase the risk of prosthesis failure. The University of California Los Angeles Activity Rating Scale is a peer-validated instrument in determining appropriate postarthroplasty activity levels (**Table 3**).[38] Variables such as male gender, lower body mass index, younger age, and higher level of preoperative activity have been associated with a higher University of California Los Angeles score postoperatively.[39] Activities such as jogging or high-impact sports should be discouraged owing to the higher risk of prosthesis failure (**Table 4**).[40] Prehabilitation may improve postoperative function and pain in some

Table 2
Commonly prescribed medications and possible impact on exercise performance

Medication	Exercise Performance	Explanations
Nonselective beta-blockers	Reduce tolerance to exercise, increase predisposition to hyperthermia, exacerbation of exercise-induced bronchospasm or asthma, impairment of left ventricular function during exercise, reduction in beta-2–stimulated glycogenesis, and reduction of Vo_2 max.[14]	Nonselective beta-blockers such as propranolol can reduce tolerance to exercise by causing reduction in beta-2–stimulated glycogenesis, producing earlier fatigue and lactate threshold. They can also increase predisposition to hyperthermia during exercise and can potentially exacerbate exercise-induced bronchospasm or asthma.[17]
Thiazides	Muscle cramping, arrhythmias, and rhabdomyolysis, hypokalemia.[14]	Thiazides can produce urinary loss of potassium and magnesium, increasing the risk of muscle cramping, arrhythmias, and rhabdomyolysis, especially during warm weather. Converting enzyme inhibitors, calcium channel blockers, alpha blockers, and central alpha agonists are medications with the least potential for negative effects on exercise performance.[18]
Statins	Fatigue, joint pain, decrease muscle strength, myalgia.[14]	Statins may induce muscle weakness, increase fatigue, and alter energy metabolism during exercise.[19] Statins may also contribute to myopathy in several ways, including reducing cholesterol for sarcolemma, endoplasmic reticular, and membrane stability, decreasing levels of coenzyme Q10, which are required for mitochondrial respiration and energy production in the muscle, and by reducing the activity of certain genes in charge of muscle repair.[20]
Metformin	Tachycardia during exercise, increase levels of lactate.[14]	Metformin can increase heart rate and lactate concentrations during exercise. However, there is new evidence in animal models that metformin was able to enhance mitochondrial respiration in skeletal muscle after just 2 wk of treatment, and thus improve exercise performance.[21]
Quinolones Steroids	Tendinitis, tendon ruptures.[14] Tendon ruptures.[14]	Quinolones and steroids increase the risk of tendinitis and tendon ruptures.[22]

(continued on next page)

Table 2 (continued)		
Medication	**Exercise Performance**	**Explanations**
PPIs	Muscle cramps, muscle weakness, arrhythmias and lethargy	PPIs, when used over long periods, have been recognized to cause muscle cramps, muscle weakness, arrhythmias and lethargy, mainly owing to hypomagnesemia.[23]
Antihistamines SSRIs	Reduce reaction time and visual discrimination Increased risk for falls, rhabdomyolysis[27]	Antihistamines and SSRIs can increase reaction time and decrease visual discrimination thereby increasing the risk for falls in older adults.[24,25] However, further studies are needed to determine the directionality of causation with greater evidentiary probity regarding the documented association between SSRIs and falls.[26]
NSAIDs	Reduce inflammation associated with exercise and improved strength recovery (only short term: <1 mo).[14]	NSAIDs have been shown to reduce the inflammation associated with exercise and improve strength recovery. Nevertheless, the side effects associated with NSAIDs in older adults (gastrointestinal bleeding and renal insufficiency) restrict their use in the long term (>1 mo).[28,29]

Abbreviations: NSAIDs, nonsteroidal anti-inflammatory drugs; PPIs, proton pump inhibitors; SSRIs, selective serotonin reuptake inhibitors.

patients undergoing joint replacement surgery, but does not significantly impact duration of stay, quality of life, or cost.[41]

BENEFITS OF EXERCISE
Physiologic Benefits of Exercise and Primary Prevention

Studies show major physiologic benefits accrue to older adults that exercise regularly (**Table 5**).[3,14,42] Although limited ability or health conditions may prohibit an older adult from performing exercise at an optimal intensity, evidence suggest that even lesser amounts of physical activity offers some health benefits.[1,3]

Social Benefits of Exercise for Older Adults

Household-based exercise is associated with social isolation among older adults.[72,73] Meanwhile, older adults who do exercise in "sports clubs" have lower rates of disability and functional decline. For example, in a study done in Japan, they followed 13,310 individuals over a period of 4 years, and showed that older adults who did exercise while participating in a sports organization did better in terms of functional decline when compared with those who did exercise by themselves. Therefore, exercise that promotes healthier social networks and social support may have additional benefits beyond the physiologic response among older adults.[74,75]

Table 3	
University of California Los Angeles table of activity	
	Check One Box That Best Describes Current Activity Level
1	Wholly inactive, dependent on others, and cannot leave residence
2	Mostly inactive or restricted to minimum activities of daily living
3	Sometimes participates in mild activities, such as walking, limited housework, and limited shopping
4	Regularly participates in mild activities
5	Sometimes participates in moderate activities, such as swimming or could do unlimited housework or shopping
6	Regularly participates in moderate activities
7	Regularly participates in active events such as bicycling
8	Regularly participates in active events, such as golf or bowling
9	Sometimes participates in impact sports, such as jogging, tennis, skiing, acrobatics, ballet, heavy labor, or backpacking
10	Regularly participates in impact sports

Data from Zahiri CA, Schmalzried TP, Szuszczewicz ES, et al. Assessing activity in joint replacement patients. J Arthroplasty 1998;13:890–5.

EXERCISE AND COMMON CHRONIC CONDITIONS

Older adults with chronic conditions should understand whether and how their condition affects their ability to do regular exercise safely (**Table 6**).[3] For sedentary older adults or for those with several medical conditions, plans should include appropriate types of activities and ways to progress at a safe and steady pace.

EXERCISE ASSESSMENT, PRESCRIPTION, AND COUNSELING

The *Go4Life* campaign's *Exercise & Physical Activity: Your Everyday Guide from the National Institute on Aging!* is an education resource for patients that can also serve

Table 4	
Activity after total hip and knee arthroplasty	
Recommended	**Not Recommended**
Bowling	High-impact aerobics
Stationary cycling	Basketball
Road cycling	Football
Ballroom dancing	Gymnastics
Low-impact aerobics	Jogging
Normal walking	Racquetball
Speed walking	Squash
Hiking	Soccer
Swimming	Volleyball
Golf	
Doubles tennis	
Canoeing	

Data from Healy WL, Iorio R, Lemos MJ. Athletic activity after joint replacement. Am J Sports Med 2001;29(3):377–88; and Healy WL, Sharma S, Schwartz B, et al. Athletic activity after total joint arthroplasty. J Bone Joint Surg Am 2008;90(10):2245–52.

Table 5
Health benefits of exercise for older adults

Overall Benefits for Older Adults

- Improves quality of life and well-being: Physical activity has positive effects for physical, social and emotional quality of life.[12,42]
- Reduces all-cause mortality risk: A sedentary person has a risk of dying almost 50 times higher than one who exercises about 5 times a week. Adherence to physical activity that burns more than 1000 Kcal/wk is associated with up to 30% reduction in all-cause mortality.[5]
- Reduces cancer risk: It also reduces overall cancer risk, including risks for breast and colon cancers by 30% and 10%, respectively.[43]
- Reduces risk of falls: Multicomponent exercise programs that include strength, balance, and endurance and last more than 6 mo are more likely to reduce the risk of falls.[44]

Specific Health Benefits	
Physiologic Benefits[14]	**Primary Prevention**
Cardiovascular and pulmonary systems	
Increased heart rate variability; better endothelial reactivity; lower inflammatory markers; reduced arterial stiffness, improved cardiac output; less atherosclerotic disease; enhanced microvasculature; improved gas exchange; stronger respiratory muscle; improves muscle function and adaptation to oxidative stress[45]; may improve function of mitochondria in the skeletal muscle[46]; improves vascularization.[47]	• Reduces cardiovascular disease risk.[48] • Reduces the risk of heart failure.[49,50] • Reduces risk of heart attack.[51] • Reduces the risk of peripheral vascular disease.[52] • Reduces high blood pressure.[53] • Lowers LDL and total cholesterol.[54] • Reduces risk of stroke[55] and recurrent stroke.[56]
Neurologic and neuropsychological systems	
Faster nerve conduction; improved balance; improved memory, attention and reaction time by increasing the size of the hippocampus and cortical volumes[57]; improved visual-spatial orientation and proprioception; improved sleep.[58]	• Reduces the risk of dementia.[59,60] • Prevents mild cognitive decline.[61] • Improves memory function.[57] • Physical inactivity is among the top reversible risk factors for Alzheimer's disease (which also included hypertension, obesity and diabetes).[62]
Immune and endocrine systems	
Reduce markers of systemic inflammation; increased basal metabolic rate; improved lipid profiles; lower body fat percentage[63]; improved insulin sensitivity and glucose homeostasis.[64–67]	• Reduces risk of obesity-related conditions.[63] • Reduces risk of diabetes mellitus.[64–67]
Musculoskeletal	
Increases muscle mass, strength, and power; preserves and increases bone mass; improves and maintains joint range of movement and flexibility[68]; increases synthesis of collagen in ligaments and tendons.	• Reduces risk of osteoporosis and risk of osteoporotic fracture, especially among postmenopausal women.[69] • Reduces risk of sarcopenia and frailty syndrome.[70,71] • Reduces age-related loss of muscle mass and improves muscle mass and strength, and physical function.[70,71]

Abbreviation: LDL, low-density lipoprotein.

Table 6
Exercise prescription and common chronic conditions

Chronic Conditions and Exercise Benefits	Exercise Prescription Guidelines
Arthritis/musculoskeletal pain (includes back pain). • Pain reduction and physical function improvement.[76]	• Land- or aquatic-based physical activity; • Aerobic training 3 to 5 times per week and resistance training 2 to 3 times per week; • Aerobic exercises (eg, walking or cycling), lower extremity strengthening exercises, tai chi, yoga,[77] and aquatic exercises (eg, aerobics, strength training performed in a therapeutic/heated indoor pool) can all alleviate pain and improve function in patients with osteoarthritis.[78]

Cardiovascular disease (includes peripheral vascular disease and heart failure)
• Improves vascularization, possibly decreasing artery stiffness and improving blood flow.[47]
	• For peripheral vascular occlusive disease, patients may need to exercise to the limits of pain tolerance each session to extend time to claudication.[78]
	• Stress testing and cardiology evaluation is recommended before vigorous exercise training in persons with known cardiovascular disease.[78,79]
	• Relevant contraindications[a,b,80]
	  ○ Absolute contraindications: Recent acute ischemic event; unstable angina; uncontrolled heart failure; symptomatic/severe aortic stenosis; uncontrolled cardiac arrhythmia; acute pulmonary embolism; acute pericarditis; suspected or known dissecting aneurysm; acute systemic infection.
	  ○ Relative (clinical) contraindications: Left main coronary artery stenosis; moderate stenotic valvular heart disease; severe arterial hypertension; hypertrophic cardiomyopathy; high-degree atrioventricular block; ventricular aneurysm; uncontrolled electrolyte imbalance; uncontrolled metabolic disease; mental or physical impairment that limits ability to exercise safely.
	  ○ Relative (situational) contraindications: Ongoing work up for cardiovascular or pulmonary disease; ongoing work up for malignancy; ongoing evaluation and treatment of pain.

Diabetes mellitus • Improves insulin resistance and glycemic control.[65,66,81] • Reduces physical impairment.[78] • Enhances weight control.[78]	• Aerobic training at least 3 d per week with no more than 2 consecutive days between bouts of activity (ie, 150 min per week of moderate to vigorous activities), and • Resistance training at moderate to vigorous intensity at least twice per week on nonconsecutive days.[82] • If the individual is using insulin or insulin secretagogues, decrease the medication doses before, during, and after exercise, and/or ingest carbohydrates if preexercise blood glucose levels are less than 100 mg/dL (5.6 mmol/L).[78]
Mental health, includes insomnia • Improves self-sleep quality, increasing sleep duration up to 1.25 h[58] • Improves depression and decrease the severity of symptoms.[83]	• Standard exercise guidelines for older adults (see **Table 1**).

(continued on next page)

Table 6 (*continued*)	
Chronic Conditions and Exercise Benefits	**Exercise Prescription Guidelines**
Osteoporosis • Preserves and improves bone loss.[84,85] • Reduces the risk of falls.[79,84,85]	• Most evidence supports resistance exercises; some evidence supports high-intensity and high-impact aerobic exercises.[78] • Add balance training to prevent falls for those with severe osteoporosis, who should avoid forward flexion exercises, using heavy weights, or side-bending exercises, because pushing, pulling, lifting, and bending exert compressive forces on the spine that may lead to fracture.[86] • Individuals with previous vertebral fractures are at risk of further vertebral fractures. It may be beneficial to consult with physical medicine and rehabilitation physicians.[78]
Falls • With balance and strength training, reduces falls and fall-related injuries.[87,88] • Reduces fear of falling.[87]	• For patients at risk of falls, balance exercises are recommended for fall prevention.[79] • Additional effective fall prevention programs are multifaceted interventions that include gait training and strength training, tai chi, Otago Exercise Program, and Stepping On.[70,89] • Patients who have problems with balance or demonstrate frailty may need to be enrolled in an observed physical therapy program and/or encouraged to be as physically active as their abilities or conditions allow.[14]
Obesity • Improves physical function.[63] • Modest weight loss.[63] • Improves quality of life.[12,42,63]	• Aerobic exercises contribute to energy expenditure to induce caloric deficit.[78] • Resistance exercises are recommended during weight loss period to help maintain lean muscle and bone mineral density.[78]
Cognitive issues • Improves cognitive function.[90] • Reduces progression to dementia.[57]	• Standard exercise guidelines for older adults (see **Table 1**), and/or tai chi.[91]
Sarcopenia and frailty syndrome • Improves muscle mass and strength.[71,92] • Improves physical function.[71,92]	• Aerobic exercise: Moderate to vigorous activity enough to raise the pulse rate to 70%–80% of the maximum heart rate. Activity performed for a minimum of 20–30 min at least 3 d/wk[93] • Resistance exercise: The progressive resistance program should involve all major muscle groups of the upper and lower extremities and trunk. One set of 8–10 different exercise, with 10–15 repetitions per set, performed on 2–3 nonconsecutive days per week. Moderate-high intensity training is recommended, in which moderate intensity is 5 or 6 on a 0–10 scale.[93] • Flexibility and balance exercise: Stretching to the point of tightness and holding the position for a few seconds. Flexibility activities are performed on all days that aerobic or muscle strengthening activity is performed. Balance training exercise 2–3 times per week.[93]

(*continued on next page*)

Table 6 *(continued)*	
Chronic Conditions and Exercise Benefits	**Exercise Prescription Guidelines**
Pulmonary diseases • Improves cardiorespiratory fitness.[47] • Decreased dyspnea and improvement in respiratory muscle function.[94]	• Exercise training is a part of the pulmonary rehabilitation program (usually 6–12 wk) for patients with chronic obstructive pulmonary disease.[78] • Exercise sessions should be timed to coincide with bronchodilator medication peak; use oxygen during exercise as needed.[78]

[a] These contraindications are based on known concerns related to cardiologic stress testing. For patients with cardiovascular disease, cardiac rehabilitation, other specialized interventions, and/or referral to specialists in the field (eg, cardiologist, exercise physiologist) may be warranted.
[b] Ongoing work should be completed before prescribing exercise in case the workup yields an unknown absolute contraindication. With regard to pain, it can be best to hold exercise until the pain is better controlled to avoid confusing etiology with exacerbating factors.

as a model for health counseling.[95] Physicians are encouraged to use the worksheets in the guide, or ones like them, for exercise prescription and counseling.

SUMMARY

The current prevalence of inactivity in older adults is unacceptable, and represents a public health problem likely to grow in concurrence with an increasing and aging populations. A challenge for health care professionals is to successfully integrate regular physical activity into patient care plans and counseling, and to collaborate with partners to support physical activity opportunities for patients.[1,3] As one of the most trusted health care professionals, physicians have an important role to play in reducing the prevalence of inactivity and fostering regular exercise among older adults.

ACKNOWLEDGMENTS

The authors thank Troy Stefano, PhD, for editorial support.

REFERENCES

1. Watson KB, Carlson SA, Gunn JP, et al. Physical inactivity among adults aged 50 years and older — United States, 2014. MMWR Morb Mortal Wkly Rep 2016;65:954–8.
2. Ward BW, Schiller JS, Goodman RA. Multiple chronic conditions among US adults: a 2012 update. Prev Chronic Dis 2014;11:130389.
3. US Department of Health and Human Services. 2008 physical activity guidelines for Americans. Washington, DC: US Department of Health and Human Services; 2008. Available at: https://health.gov/paguidelines/pdf/paguide.pdf.
4. Centers for Disease Control and Prevention. Behavioral risk factor surveillance system. Available at: http://www.cdc.gov/nccdphp/brfss. Accessed May 24, 2017.
5. Lee IM, Skerrett PJ. Physical activity and all-cause mortality: what is the dose-response relation? Med Sci Sports Exerc 2001;33(6 Suppl):S459–71 [discussion: S493–4].
6. Abramson S, Stein J, Schaufele M, et al. Personal exercise habits and counseling practices of primary care physicians: a national survey. Clin J Sport Med 2000;10(1):40–8.

7. AuYoung M, Linke SE, Pagoto S, et al. Integrating physical activity in primary care practice. Am J Med 2016;129(10):1022–9.
8. Belza B. The PRC-HAN Physical Activity Conference Planning Workgroup (2007). Moving ahead: strategies and tools to plan, conduct, and maintain effective community-based physical activity programs for older adults. Atlanta (GA): Centers for Disease Control and Prevention. Available at: https://www.cdc.gov/aging/pdf/community-based_physical_activity_programs_for_older_adults.pdf. Accessed August 8, 2017.
9. Secretary's Advisory Committee on Health Promotion and Disease Prevention Objectives for 2020. Healthy people 2020: an opportunity to address the societal determinants of health in the United States. July 26, 2010. Available at: http://www.healthypeople.gov/2010/hp2020/advisory/SocietalDeterminantsHealth.htm. Accessed June 2, 2017.
10. Powell LM, Slater S, Chaloupka FJ, et al. Availability of physical activity–related facilities and neighborhood demographic and socioeconomic characteristics: a national study. Am J Public Health 2006;96(9):1676–80.
11. Centers for Disease Control and Prevention (CDC). The state of aging and health in America — 2013. Atlanta (GA): CDC, US Dept. of Health and Human Services; 2013. Available at: https://www.cdc.gov/aging/pdf/state-aging-health-in-america-2013.pdf.
12. Valencia WM, Stoutenberg M, Florez H. Weight loss and physical activity for disease prevention in obese older adults: an important role for lifestyle management. Curr Diab Rep 2014;14(10):539.
13. Nelson ME, Rejeski WJ, Blair SN, et al. Physical activity and public health in older adults: recommendation from the American College of Sports Medicine and the American Heart Association. Circulation 2007;116:1094–105.
14. Mora JC, Ciocon J. Elder care - A resource for interprofessional providers: physical exercise guidelines for older adults. portal of geriatrics online education; 2013. Available at: http://www.pogoe.org/productid/21715. Accessed June 2, 2017.
15. Kantor ED, Rehm CD, Haas JS, et al. Trends in prescription drug use among adults in the United States from 1999-2012. JAMA 2015;314(17):1818–31.
16. Merck Institute of Aging and Health (MIAH) and Centers for Disease Control and Prevention (CDC). The State of aging and health in America 2004. Washington, DC; Atlanta (GA): MIAH; CDC, US Dept. of Health and Human Services; 2004. Available at: https://www.cdc.gov/aging/pdf/state_of_aging_and_health_in_america_2004.pdf. Accessed June 2, 2017.
17. Gullestad L, Hallen J, Medbø, et al. The effect of acute vs chronic treatment with beta-adrenoceptor blockade on exercise performance, haemodynamic and metabolic parameters in healthy men and women. Br J Clin Pharmacol 1996;41:57–67.
18. Chick TW, Halperin AK, Gacek EM. The effect of antihypertensive medications on exercise performance: a review. Med Sci Sports Exerc 1988;20(5):447–54.
19. Parker BA, Capizzi JA, Grimaldi AS, et al. The effect of statins on skeletal muscle function. Circulation 2013;127(1):96–103.
20. Deichmann RE, Lavie CJ, Asher T, et al. The interaction between statins and exercise: mechanisms and strategies to counter the musculoskeletal side effects of this combination therapy. Ochsner J 2015;15(4):429–37. Available at: https://www.ncbi.nlm.nih.gov/pmc/articles/PMC4679305/pdf/i1524-5012-15-4-429.pdf. Accessed June 2, 2017.

21. Kristensen JM, Larsen S, Helge JW, et al. Two weeks of metformin treatment en-hances mitochondrial respiration in skeletal muscle of AMPK kinase dead but not wild type mice. PLoS One 2013;8(1):e53533.
22. Arabyat RM, Raisch DW, McKoy JM, et al. Fluoroquinolone-associated tendon-rupture: a summary of reports in the Food and Drug Administration's adverse event reporting system. Expert Opin Drug Saf 2015;14(11):1653–60.
23. Toh JWT, Ong E, Wilson R. Hypomagnesaemia associated with long-term use of proton pump inhibitors. Gastroenterol Rep (Oxf) 2015;3(3):243–53.
24. Montgomery LC, Deuster PA. Effects of antihistamine medications on exercise performance. Implications for sportspeople. Sports Med 1993;15(3):179–95.
25. Marcum ZA, Perera S, Thorpe JM, et al. Antidepressant use and recurrent falls in community-dwelling older adults: findings from the Health ABC Study. Ann Pharmacother 2016;50(7):525–33.
26. Gebara MA, Lipsey KL, Karp JK, et al. Cause or effect? selective serotonin reup-take inhibitors and falls in older adults: a systematic review. Am J Geriatr Psychi-atry 2015;23(10):1016–28.
27. Snyder M, Kish T. Sertraline-induced rhabdomyolysis: a case report and literature review. Am J Ther 2016;23(2):e561–5.
28. Baldwin AC, Stevenson SW, Dudley GA. Nonsteroidal anti-inflammatory therapy after eccentric exercise in healthy older individuals. J Gerontol A Biol Sci Med Sci 2001;56(8):M510–3.
29. Jankowski CM, Shea K, Barry DW, et al. Timing of ibuprofen use and musculo-skeletal adaptations to exercise training in older adults. Bone Rep 2015;1:1–8.
30. Coleman-Jensen A, Rabbitt MP, Gregory CA, et al. Household food security in the United States in 2015, ERR-215. Washington, DC: U.S. Department of Agricul-ture, Economic Research Service; 2016. Available at: https://www.ers.usda.gov/webdocs/publications/79761/err-215.pdf?v=42636. Accessed June 2, 2017.
31. Manore MM. Effect of physical activity on thiamine, riboflavin, and vitamin B-6 re-quirements. Am J Clin Nutr 2000;72(2 Suppl):598S–606S. Available at: http://ajcn.nutrition.org/content/72/2/598s.long. Accessed June 2, 2017.
32. Rodriguez NR, DiMarco NM, Langley S. Position of the American Dietetic Association, Dietitians of Canada, and the American College of Sports Medicine: nutrition and athletic performance. J Am Diet Assoc 2009;109(3):509–27 [Erratum appears in J Am Diet Assoc 2013;113(12):1759].
33. Sawka MN, Burke LM, Eichner ER, et al, American College of Sports Medicine. American College of Sports Medicine position stand. Exercise and fluid replace-ment. Med Sci Sports Exerc 2007;39(2):377–90.
34. Chen AL, Mears SC, Hawkins RJ. Orthopaedic care of the aging athlete. J Am Acad Orthop Surg 2005;13(6):407–16.
35. Hootman JM, Macera CA, Ainsworth BE, et al. Predictors of lower extremity injury among recreationally active adults. Clin J Sport Med 2002;12:99–106.
36. Little RM, Paterson DH, Humphreys DA, et al. A 12-month incidence of exercise-related injuries in previously sedentary community-dwelling older adults following an exercise intervention. BMJ Open 2013;3(6):e002831.
37. Kannus P, Niittymäki S, Järvinen M, et al. Sports injuries in elderly athletes: a three-year prospective, controlled study. Age Ageing 1989;18(4):263–70.
38. Terwee CB, Bouwmeester W, van Elsland SL, et al. Instruments to assess physical activity in patients with osteoarthritis of the hip or knee: a systematic review of measurement properties. Osteoarthritis Cartilage 2011;19(6):620–33.
39. Williams DH, Greidanus NV, Masri BA, et al. Predictors of participation in sports after hip and knee arthroplasty. Clin Orthop Relat Res 2012;470(2):555–61.

40. Malcolm TL, Szubski CR, Nowacki AS, et al. Activity levels and functional outcomes of young patients undergoing total hip arthroplasty. Orthopedics 2014; 37(11):e983–92.
41. Wang L, Lee M, Zhang Z, et al. Does preoperative rehabilitation for patients planning to undergo joint replacement surgery improve outcomes? A systematic review and meta-analysis of randomised controlled trials. BMJ Open 2016;6(2): e009857.
42. Gill DL, Hammond CC, Reifsteck EJ, et al. Physical activity and quality of life. J Prev Med Public Health 2013;46(Suppl 1):S28–34.
43. Thune I, Furberg AS. Physical activity and cancer risk: dose-response and cancer, all sites and site-specific. Med Sci Sports Exerc 2001;33(6 Suppl):S530–50 [discussion: S609–10].
44. Cadore EL, Rodríguez-Mañas L, Sinclair A, et al. Effects of different exercise interventions on risk of falls, gait ability, and balance in physically frail older adults: a systematic review. Rejuvenation Res 2013;16(2):105–14.
45. Gibala MJ, Little JP, van Essen M, et al. Short-term sprint interval versus traditional endurance training: similar initial adaptations in human skeletal muscle and exercise performance. J Physiol 2006;575(3):901–11.
46. Cobley JN, Mount PR, Burniston JG, et al. Exercise improves mitochondrial and redox-regulated stress responses in the elderly: better late than never! Biogerontology 2015;16:249–64.
47. Rakobowchuk M, Tanguay S, Burgomaster KA, et al. Sprint interval and traditional endurance training induce similar improvements in peripheral arterial stiffness and flow-mediated dilation in healthy humans. Am J Physiol Regul Integr Comp Physiol 2008;295:R236–42.
48. Hussain SR, Macaluso A, Pearson SJ. High-intensity interval training versus moderate-intensity continuous training in the prevention/management of cardiovascular disease. Cardiol Rev 2016;24:273–81.
49. Davies EJ, Moxham T, Rees K, et al. Exercise training for systolic heart failure: Cochrane systematic review and meta-analysis. Eur J Heart Fail 2010;12:706–15.
50. Taylor RS, Sagar VA, Davies EJ, et al. Exercise-based rehabilitation for heart failure. Cochrane Database Syst Rev 2014;(4):CD003331.
51. Yusuf S, Hawken S, Ounpuu S, et al, INTERHEART Study Investigators. Effect of potentially modifiable risk factors associated with myocardial infarction in 52 countries (INTERHEART study): case-control study. Lancet 2004;364(9438): 937–52.
52. Foley TR, Armstrong EJ, Waldo SW. Contemporary evaluation and management of lower extremity peripheral artery disease. Heart 2016;102:1436–41.
53. Diaz KM, Shimbo D. Physical activity and the prevention of hypertension. Curr Hypertens Rep 2013;15(6):659–68.
54. Myers J. Exercise and cardiovascular health. Circulation 2003;107:2e–5.
55. Goldstein LB, Bushnell CD, Adams RJ, et al. Guidelines for the primary prevention of stroke: a guideline for healthcare professionals from the American Heart Association/American Stroke Association. Stroke 2011;42:517–84.
56. Furie KL, Kasner SE, Adams RJ, et al. Guidelines for the prevention of stroke in patients with stroke or transient ischemic attack: a guideline for healthcare professionals from the American Heart Association/American Stroke Association. Stroke 2011;42:227–76.
57. Erickson KI, Voss MW, Prakash RS, et al. Exercise training increases size of hippocampus and improves memory. Proc Natl Acad Sci U S A 2011;108(7): 3017–22.

58. Reid KJ, Baron KG, Lu B, et al. Aerobic exercise improves self-reported sleep and quality of life in older adults with insomnia. Sleep Med 2010;11(9):934–40.
59. Hamer M, Chida Y. Physical activity and risk of neurodegenerative disease: a systematic review of prospective evidence. Psychol Med 2009;39:3–11.
60. Guure CB, Ibrahim NA, Adam MB, et al. Impact of physical activity on cognitive decline, dementia, and its subtypes: meta-analysis of prospective studies. Biomed Res Int 2017;2017:9016924.
61. Sattler C, Erickson KI, Toro P, et al. Physical fitness as a protective factor for cognitive impairment in a prospective population-based study in Germany. J Alzheimers Dis 2011;26:709–18.
62. Norton S, Matthews FE, Barnes DE, et al. Potential for primary prevention of Alzheimer's disease: an analysis of population-based data. Lancet Neurol 2014;13: 788–94.
63. Valencia WM, Sood R. Obesity and weight gain in older persons. In: Pachana NA, editor. Encyclopedia of geropsychology. Springer; 2016. Available at: https://www.researchgate.net/publication/303860308_Obesity_and_Weight_Gain_in_Older_People. Accessed May 5, 2017.
64. Valencia WM, Florez H. Endocrinology and metabolism. In: Burton J, Lee A, Potter J, editors. Geriatrics for specialists. Springer; 2017. p. 269–82.
65. Valencia WM, Florez H. Pharmacological treatment of diabetes in older people. Diabetes Obes Metab 2014;16(12):1192–203.
66. Valencia WM, Florez HJ. How to prevent the microvascular complications of type 2 diabetes beyond glucose control. BMJ 2017;356:i6505.
67. Davis N, Ma Y, Delahanty LM, et al. Predictors of sustained reduction in energy and fat intake in the Diabetes Prevention Program Outcomes Study intensive lifestyle intervention. J Acad Nutr Diet 2013;113:1455–64.
68. Garber CE, Blissmer B, Deschenes MR, et al. American College of Sports Medicine position stand. Quantity and quality of exercise for developing and maintaining cardiorespiratory, musculoskeletal, and neuromotor fitness in apparently healthy adults: guidance for prescribing exercise. Med Sci Sports Exerc 2011; 43(7):1334–59.
69. Howe TE, Shea B, Dawson LJ, et al. Exercise for preventing and treating osteoporosis in postmenopausal women. Cochrane Database Syst Rev 2011;(7):CD000333.
70. Kim HK, Suzuki T, Saito K, et al. Long-term effects of exercise and amino acid supplementation on muscle mass, physical function and falls in community-dwelling elderly Japanese sarcopenic women: a 4-year follow-up study. Geriatr Gerontol Int 2016;16:175–81.
71. Crane JD, Macneil LG, Tarnopolsky MA. Long-term aerobic exercise is associated with greater muscle strength throughout the life span. J Gerontol A Biol Sci Med Sci 2013;68:631–8.
72. Holt-Lunstad J, Smith TB, Layton JB. Social relationships and mortality risk: a meta-analytic review. PLoS Med 2010;7(7):e1000316.
73. Robins LM, Hill KD, Finch CF, et al. The association between physical activity and social isolation in community-dwelling older adults. Aging Ment Health 2016;1–8. https://doi.org/10.1080/13607863.2016.1242116.
74. Kanamori S, Kai Y, Aida J, et al, JAGES Group. Social participation and the prevention of functional disability in older Japanese: the JAGES cohort study. PLoS One 2014;9(6):e99638.
75. Keyes CL, Michalec B, Kobau R, et al. Social support and health-related quality of life among older adults. MMWR Morb Mortal Wkly Rep 2005;54(17):433–7.

Available at: https://www.cdc.gov/mmwr/preview/mmwrhtml/mm5417a4.htm. Accessed June 2, 2017.

76. Koltyn KF. Using physical activity to manage pain in older adults. J Aging Phys Act 2002;10(2):226–39.

77. Cheung C, Wyman JF, Resnick B, et al. Yoga for managing knee osteoarthritis in older women: a pilot randomized controlled trial. BMC Complement Altern Med 2014;14(1):160.

78. Lee PG, Jackson EA, Richardson CR. Exercise prescriptions in older adults. Am Fam Physician 2017;95(7):425–32.

79. Chodzko-Zajko WJ, Proctor DN, Fiatarone Singh MA, et al. American College of Sports Medicine position stand. Exercise and physical activity for older adults. Med Sci Sports Exerc 2009;41(7):1510–30.

80. Fletcher GF, Ades PA, Kligfield P, et al. Exercise standards for testing and training: a scientific statement from the American Heart Association. Circulation 2013;128:873–934.

81. Valencia WM. Preventing hypoglycemia in the older adult with diabetes. Geriatric Fast Facts #65. Available at: http://www.geriatricfastfacts.com/fast-facts/preventing-hypoglycemia-older-adult-diabetes. Accessed June 2, 2017.

82. Colberg SR, Albright AL, Blissmer BJ, et al. Exercise and type 2 diabetes: American College of Sports Medicine and the American Diabetes Association: joint position statement. Med Sci Sports Exerc 2010;42(12):2282–303.

83. Bridle C, Spanjers K, Patel S, et al. Effect of exercise on depression severity in older people: systematic review and meta-analysis of randomised controlled trials. Br J Psychiatry 2012;201:180–5.

84. U.S. Preventive Services Task Force. Screening for osteoporosis: U.S. Preventive Services Task Force recommendation statement. Ann Intern Med 2011;154(5):356–64.

85. Diab DL, Watts NB. Diagnosis and treatment of osteoporosis in older adults. Endocrinol Metab Clin North Am 2013;42(2):305–17.

86. Watts NB, Bilezikian JP, Camacho PM, et al. American Association of Clinical Endocrinologists medical guidelines for clinical practice for the diagnosis and treatment of postmenopausal osteoporosis. Endocr Pract 2010;16(Suppl 3):1–37.

87. Kendrick D, Kumar A, Carpenter H, et al. Exercise for reducing fear of falling in older people living in the community. Cochrane Database Syst Rev 2014;(11):CD009848.

88. Gillespie LD, Robertson M, Gillespie WJ, et al. Interventions for preventing falls in older people living in the community. Cochrane Database Syst Rev 2012;(9):CD007146.

89. Stevens JA, Burns E. A CDC compendium of effective fall interventions: what works for community-dwelling older adults. 3rd edition. Atlanta (GA): Centers for Disease Control and Prevention, National Center for Injury Prevention and Control; 2015. Available at: https://www.cdc.gov/homeandrecreationalsafety/falls/compendium.html.

90. Cai H, Li G, Hua S, et al. Effect of exercise on cognitive function in chronic disease patients: a meta-analysis and systematic review of randomized controlled trials. Clin Interv Aging 2017;11:773–83.

91. Wayne PM, Walsh JN, Taylor-Piliae RE, et al. The impact of Tai Chi on cognitive performance in older adults: a systematic review and meta-analysis. J Am Geriatr Soc 2014;62(1):25–39.

92. Lozano-Montoya I, Correa-Pérez A, Abraha I, et al. Nonpharmacological interventions to treat physical frailty and sarcopenia in older patients: a systematic overview - the SENATOR Project ONTOP Series. Clin Interv Aging 2017;12:721–40.
93. Aguirre LE, Villareal DT. Physical exercise as therapy for frailty. Nestle Nutr Inst Workshop Ser 2015;83:83–92.
94. Spruit MA, Burtin C, De Boever P, et al. COPD and exercise: does it make a difference? Breathe (Sheff) 2016;12(2):e38–49.
95. US Department of Health and Human Services: National Institute on Aging. Exercise & physical activity: your everyday guide from the National Institute on Aging! Gaithersburg (MD): National Institute on Aging Information Center; 2013. No. 09-4258. Available at: https://go4life.nia.nih.gov/sites/default/files/nia_exercise_and_physical_activity.pdf. Accessed June 12, 2017.

Moving?

Make sure your subscription moves with you!

To notify us of your new address, find your **Clinics Account Number** (located on your mailing label above your name), and contact customer service at:

Email: journalscustomerservice-usa@elsevier.com

800-654-2452 (subscribers in the U.S. & Canada)
314-447-8871 (subscribers outside of the U.S. & Canada)

Fax number: 314-447-8029

Elsevier Health Sciences Division
Subscription Customer Service
3251 Riverport Lane
Maryland Heights, MO 63043

*To ensure uninterrupted delivery of your subscription, please notify us at least 4 weeks in advance of move.

Printed and bound by CPI Group (UK) Ltd, Croydon, CR0 4YY
03/10/2024
01040390-0015